YOGA
HOLISTIC
PRACTICE MANUAL

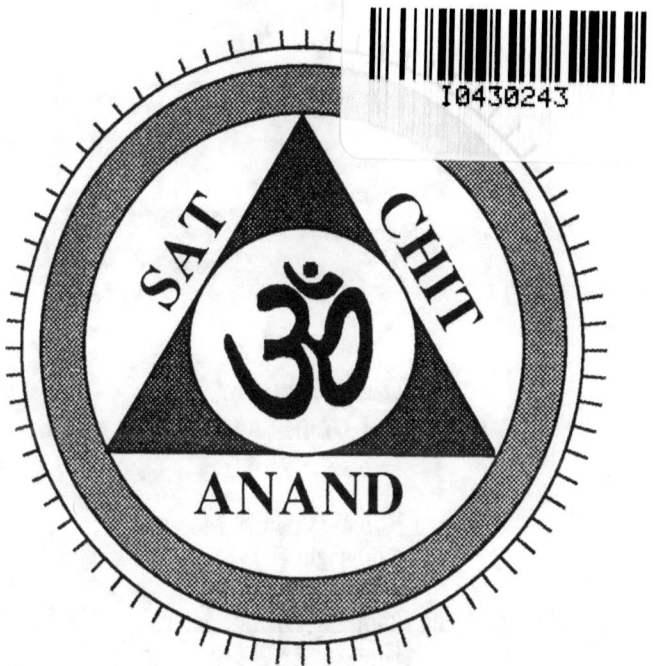

By Yogi Shanti Desai

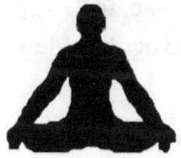

SHANTI YOGA INSTITUTE

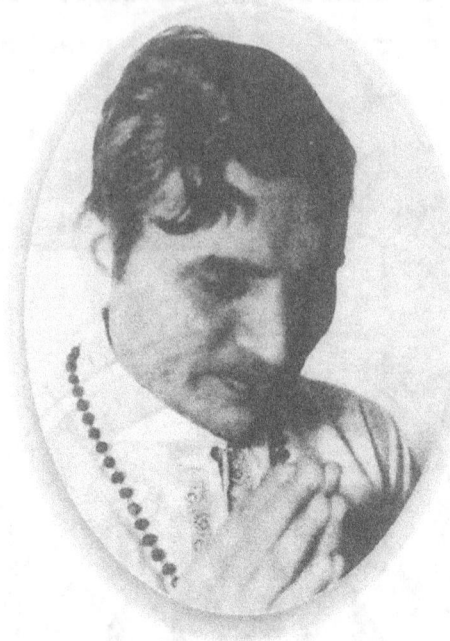

Jai Bhagwan!
I greet the Divine within you.

Yoga-Holistic Practice Manual
Copyright © 1988
Revised Printing 2004
Formerly The Complete Practice Manual of Yoga
Copyright © 1976

Yoga Retreat
943 Central Avenue, Ocean City, N.J. 08226
609-399-1974
www.yogishantidesai.com

Vegetarian Recipes - Nayana Desai
Editing - Proofreading - Sue & Marty Lutz
Typesetting and Organization - Ruth Sperber
Graphics & Charts - Harry Sperber

ISBN: 1-4635-0766-6
ISBN-13: 9781463507664

Author's Comments

The path of truth is for the brave only. Krishna teaches in the Gita that out of thousands maybe only one searches for the truth.

Temptations on the path can lead one (consciously or unconsciously) to escape by becoming a false Guru or Chela (disciple) or a combination of both.

The disciple gets trapped into fantasies of psychic phenomena, a mystical Guru, and instant enlightenment. Following the crowd he runs from group to group and teacher to teacher. He chooses his Guru based on the external facade and publicity, joining the group that gives him identity to satisfy his ego. He enjoys being manipulated by the leader and group psychology while possibly missing a simple and honest teacher available to him.

The false Guru is motivated and trapped in ambition for wealth, power, name and fame, and uses borrowed wisdom as the basis of his teaching. He pampers, controls, and manipulates his disciples, encouraging them to spread the word about his spirituality and mysticism and his selfless service, while he hides from the world and becomes inaccessible. He promises to save the world but cannot maintain peace and harmony within his own family. The false Guru's dogmas, complex philosophies and imaginary fantasies trap both himself and his disciples keeping them from real truth. These illusions and pretenses crumble in time. They do not give lasting freedom but only create confusion and burdens.

To find the truth one must open up and face reality, let go of imitations and stand on his own feet rather than try to escape by hiding from reality. One should not put on a show of spirituality. Instead, one should allow his spiritual evolution to be an internal process which expresses itself naturally through a balanced and contented life. Free your mind from dogmas and fantasies and learn to trust your inner self. Then you can experience truth as it presents itself in your life. Truth is simple and straightforward.

I have presented the aspects of Yoga in a simple, logical and scientific way without fantasy or mystery. I hope to ignite the spark of inspiration in the reader and to dispel his doubts so he can take charge of his own life in his search for truth.

Yogi Shanti Desai

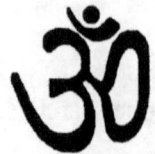 # BRAHMAN – AUM

Braham is the Universal aspect of God. Brahman is without boundaries (Anant), without qualities (Nirguna), without form (Nirakar), non-dual (Advaita), invisible (Avyakta), uninvolved and transcendental (Nishkriya). Brahman is represented as "aum", the universal vibration or primordial sound (Pranav) and represented by the above symbol. It is a mathematical expression.

3 Represents:

OMNIPOTENT – It represents the three qualities of nature (Gunas), which are responsible for creation, sustenance and dissolution. GOD G is the Generator (Brahma) O is the Operator (Vishnu) D is the Destroyer (Mahesh). Brahman transcends them all.

OMNIPRESENT – It represents the past, present and future. Brahman transcends time.

OMNISCIENT – It represents the three states of consciousness: Waking (Jagrat), Dreaming (Swapna) and Slumber (Susupti). Brahman exists in a transcendental state of consciousness (Turiya).

0 Represents:

The material universe (Jagat), which is projected from Brahman and is permeated by Brahman. Brahman is homogeneous with its creation. Jagat is impermanent, revolves in cyclical rhythm and has a value of zero from the standpoint of Brahman. It is constantly changing (Mithya).

The line connecting 3 and 0 represents the projection of Jagat from Brahman. It is also a minus sign.

The horn shape beneath the dot represents remainder existence (Shesha).

The dot above the horn represents the existence of Brahman in a microcosmic form, as individual self (Atman). Brahman is indivisible and indestructible.

Brahman is whole and its projection, Jagat, is whole. Jagat is projected during the evolution cycle and is withdrawn during the involution cycle. Brahman remains unchanged with or without Jagat. Brahman is visible in the light of knowledge, while Jagat is visible in the darkness of ignorance. Brahman is real while Jagat is unreal (Mithya). Brahman is experienced when one transcends the mind. Jagat is experienced with the mind and senses.

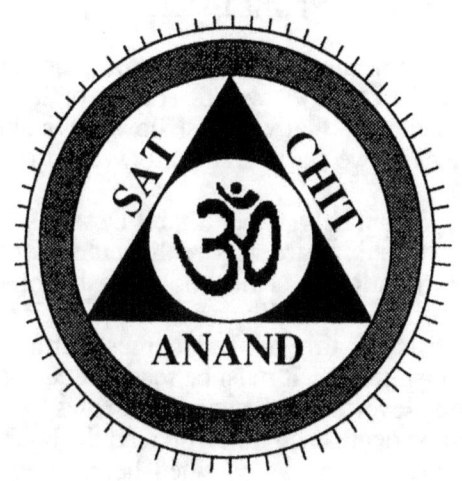

The qualities of Brahman are
SAT, CHIT & ANAND

All Living creatures are a creation of Brahman, separated from Brahman and constantly seeking union with Brahman as Sat, Chit and Anand.

SAT represents imperishable existence. One seeks immortality. When Jagat with names and forms is destroyed, Brahman still exists. When golden ornaments are destroyed, the gold remains.

CHIT represents consciousness and knowledge. One seeks knowledge to find comfort, freedom and control over life. Brahman maintains universal order through cosmic intelligence.

ANAND represents bliss. One seeks lasting happiness at all times and under all circumstances. Brahman is the inexhaustible source of bliss.

A wise person turns inward toward Self and finds fulfillment and liberation. A foolish person runs outward toward Jagat and finds frustration, bondage and suffering.

FOREWORD

With the fast pace, stress, competition, and "hurry-sickness" in today's world, sooner or later most of us come to the conclusion that we must slow down and change our lifestyle. Where do we start? What are we to do? To whom do we turn?

Fortunately, I met Shanti Desai. The example of his life and his teachings are very realistic and applicable to our current daily situations. This book has become for me an encyclopedia for living. Unlike a novel, which is read once and returned to the shelf, this book becomes a lifetime source of guidance and inspiration. It must be read with an open mind and heart. As your level of understanding grows, you will derive new meaning and depth each time you read the book.

The benefits described herein are real and will come to you in time with consistent practice. Do not force any of the disciplines, nor expect to change overnight. Rather, incorporate the teachings into your life gradually. Your life will improve in proportion to your open-mindedness, commitment, and sincerity.

Suzanne Lutz

We are all on "the path," some with more awareness than others. This book is primarily intended for the serious student. If you utilize this book as a source of understanding, as guidance in your daily practice, as inspiration, your awareness will grow. The path is never easy but confusion can be eliminated by following the teachings of a master. You will find that as your understanding evolves, that this book when read and reread, will seem like many different books providing understanding and insight at many different levels.

For those who are new to the path this book will prove interesting reading and might be the straw that breaks the camel's back of maya (illusion) and will provide the necessary motivation to lead you to question "Why am I here, what is life all about, why are things the way they are, how can I gain control of my life?"

Marty Lutz

TABLE OF CONTENTS

INTRODUCTION

1. THE MEANING AND GOAL OF YOGA........3
    ORIGIN OF YOGA.........................6
    YOGA IS A SCIENCE AND ART 6
    MANY PATHS OF YOGA 6
2. HISTORY AND EVOLUTION OF YOGA.......8

PHILOSOPHY AND PRACTICES

3. RAJA YOGA 17
    YAMA (Restrictions)........................ 18
    NIYAMA (Positive Disciplines)...................... 22
    ASANA (Position)........................ 25
    PRANAYAMA (Breathing Control).................. 26
    PRATYAHARA (Sense Withdrawal)................. 27
    DHARANA (Concentration) 27
    DHYANA (Meditation) 28
    SAMADHI (Complete Absorption) 28
    ABHYASA Persistent practice 32
    VAIRAGYA Non-attachment/Renunciation 33
4. HATHA YOGA................................ 38
    HOW SHOULD ONE PRACTICE.......................... 39
    GENERAL RULES........................ 42
    GENERAL BENEFITS OF YOGA 42
        Tension 43
        Cleansing........................ 43
        Endocrine Glands........................ 43
        Involuntary Organs........................ 44
        Back and Spine 44
        Weight and Muscle Tone 44
        Emotional Balance........................ 44
        Longevity........................ 45
5. YOGA POSITIONS 46
    GETTING READY 46
        Sleeping, Waking, Cleansing 46
        Stretching and Limbering.................. 47
    POSTURES 48
        Shoulderstand Routine.................... 48
        Head-to-Knee 48
        Bow........................ 49

	Twist	49
	Lion and Abdominal Lift	49
	Mudras	50
	Lotus-Meditation-Relaxation	50
6.	BREATHING (Pranayama)	59
	FUNCTIONS OF BREATH	59
	BREATHING MECHANISM	59
	WRONG BREATHING	60
	BEGINNER'S BREATHING	61
	YOGIC BREATHING	62
	WALKING BREATHING	63
	RHYTHMIC BREATHING	63
	RECHARGING BREATHING	64
	HEALING BREATHINGS	64
	CLEANSING BREATHINGS	66
	ANULOMA VILOMA PRANAYAMA	68
	PREPARATION FOR PRANAYAMA	71
	BENEFITS	71
7.	RELAXATION	73
	STAGES OF RELAXATION	74
	Physical Relaxation	74
	Mental Relaxation	75
	Spiritual Relaxation	75
	A TECHNIQUE OF RELAXATION	76
	BENEFITS OF RELAXATION	78
8.	KUNDALINI YOGA	79
9.	CONCENTRATION and MEDITATION	82
	EXPLANATION	82
	PREPARATION	82
	METHODS	83
10.	BHAKTI YOGA	91
	HOW TO DEVELOP BHAKTI	95
11.	MANTRA YOGA	99
	BENEFITS	100
	DIFFERENT KINDS OF MANTRAS	102
	HOW TO CHANT MANTRAS AND JAPAS	106
	USE OF MALA (ROSARY) FOR JAPA	108
	BIJA MANTRA AND OM CHANTING	108
	HOW TO CHANT OM OR AUM	110
	GURU MANTRA	111
	MAHA OR UNIVERSAL MANTRAS	115
	MISCELLANEOUS MANTRAS	116
	ARTI	117

12. SURRENDER YOGA 120
    MEDITATION TECHNIQUE..........................122
13. GURU 124
14. INITIATION (Diksha)...........................127
15. GNANA YOGA 129
    THE GNANA YOGA PATH...........................129
    SCRIPTURAL AUTHORITY 131
    OUR WORLD OF ILLUSION.........................131
    THE NATURE OF MAYA 132
    ISHVARA.......................................134
    MANIFESTATIONS 135
    BODY SHEATHS 135
    MEDITATION TECHNIQUE NO. 1 137
    MEDITATION TECHNIQUE NO. 2 138
    COSMOLOGY 140
    MACROCOSM AND MICROCOSM 142
16. REINCARNATION.................................143
    LAW OF PERMANENCE............................143
    MEMORY OF PREVIOUS LIVES.....................144
    LAW OF JUSTICE AND ORDER.....................145
    LAW OF KARMA 145
    LIFE AFTER DEATH.............................148
    FREEDOM FROM KARMA 148
    BENEFITS 149
17. KARMA YOGA 152
    THE PATH OF KARMA YOGA.......................152
    THE REWARDS OF KARMA YOGA 153
    KARMA YOGA AND DUTY 154
    SCRIPTURAL AUTHORITY 155
    JOINT FAMILY SYSTEM..........................156
    SOCIETY 158
    MARRIAGE 159

DIET

18. DIET AND NUTRITION 165
    INTRODUCTION TO DIET 165
    NUTRITION.....................................166
    ACID-ALKALINE BALANCING......................169

19. YOGA AND DIET..170
    THREE QUALITIES OF FOOD.......................170
    PRANA 171
    DIET RECOMMENDATIONS 171
    AYURVEDA..177
20. NATURAL AND HEALTH FOODS...178
    HOLISTIC HEALTH PRODUCTS 184
    MACROBIOTICS 184
    TAO - Balance of Yin and Yang....................185
21. VEGETARIANISM...............................188
    NONVIOLENCE 192
22. FASTING..194
    LONG TERM FAST 195
    SHORT TERM FAST...196
    SUGGESTIONS/RULES FOR FASTING 196
23. CLEANSING 199
    METHODS OF CLEANSING 199
24. VEGETARIAN RECIPES 204
    SOUPS...204
    RICE..207
    BREADS...209
    VEGETABLES 211
    CASSEROLES..213
    SIDE DISHES 215
    SWEETS 219

GUIDANCE

25. HATHA YOGA COURSE 225
26. DAILY PRACTICE ROUTINE 227
    YOGA POSITIONS 227
    BREATHING/MEDITATION..........................228
    DAILY DISCIPLINES...............................229
    GENERAL DISCIPLINES...........................230
27. DAILY INFLUENCE OF YOGA................231
28. AFFIRMATIONS 235
    PROCESS OF AFFIRMATION.......................235
    PREPARATION..238
    GENERAL AFFIRMATIONS 240
29. DAILY AFFIRMATIONS (7 days).............241

Y O G A

H O L I S T I C
P R A C T I C E
M A N U A L

INTRODUCTION

1. Meaning and Goal of Yoga

2. History and Evolution of Yoga

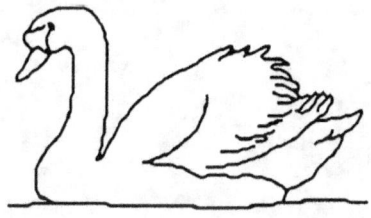

1

THE MEANING AND GOAL OF YOGA

Yoga means integration of body, mind, and spirit. Peace and harmony come in proportion to this integration. The word Yoga is derived from the Sanskrit root "Yuj" which means yoking or union. Yoga is a way of uniting the body, mind, and spirit to God (Cosmic-consciousness), or uniting the finite individual self (Jivatma) with the cosmic infinite Self (Paramatma). The practice of Yoga begins with a systematic awareness and mastery of our physical, mental, and spiritual nature. Gradually we discover our higher self as we develop our potential and bring our total being into harmony and rhythm with the universe. The definition and goal of Yoga are explained from various points of view as follows:

1. Our relationship with God is like the relationship of a drop of water to the ocean. Quantitatively they are different, but qualitatively they are the same. When the drop of water falls into the ocean, it merges and becomes the ocean. In the same way we must merge with God and become God. We are created in the image of God. We are reflections of God. How, then, can we be sinners? Yoga offers the positive and most optimistic approach that we are potentially divine and perfect. Christ taught, "Be ye therefore perfect even as thy father which is in heaven is perfect."

This perfection is not to be gained from outside. Meditation helps us discover this perfection, which is the very nature of our consciousness. This perfection will always be within us, but it is hidden by our ignorance. Ignorance is produced by the restlessness of the mind. The goal of Yoga is "Know thy Self." To know thy Self is to know our true essence (Atman) which is a witness to our physical, mental, and emotional changes. It also witnesses our waking, dreaming, dreamless sleep, and unconscious states of mind without being affected by them.

2. Yoga is a process of dehypnotism. We have hypnotized ourselves as being the physical body, limited by time, space, and causation. This process, repeated by our previous incarnations and strengthened by our daily experiences in life,

paralyzes us, and we accept these limitations and suffer the consequences. We are kings but we act as if we are beggars. Yoga reverses this process, and we awaken from this hypnotic spell feeling our existence to be pure consciousness while the body, mind, and intellect function as instruments working for us at our command.

A prince, kidnapped by some beggars when he was a baby, grew up thinking he was a beggar. When he was grown, a wise man recognized him from a birthmark and he was established as the king. When he realized his true identity, he acted like a king and not like a beggar. A baby lion grew up with a flock of sheep and acted like a sheep. He was timid, frightened of little things, and followed the other sheep without question. One day a lion saw him in the flock, pulled him aside and led him to a lake where he saw his reflection in the water. Realizing his true nature was that of a lion, he started to act like one and his life was transformed. In the same way, when a spiritual master reveals our true nature to us, our life is transformed and we are freed from the myth of limited identity with our physical body and the material world. When this hypnotic spell is removed, we experience the highest possible freedom.

God is our spiritual Father. He provides all the comforts of our life. We pray earnestly to Him while in our mother's womb for release from suffering. As soon as we are born, however, we forget Him due to the overwhelming power of maya (cosmic illusion). We denounce our Father and roam the world in search of happiness, going through various pleasant and unpleasant experiences in life. When we are suffering and rejected by the world, we remember our Father. The practice of Yoga is the journey of a prodigal son towards the home of his Father. The goal of Yoga is to be reunited with the Father and find peace and rest.

Everyone in the world (young or old, moral or immoral) is searching for this union to find ultimate freedom. We may use various means to find this freedom. It may be sensual pleasure, food, sex, wealth, power, or criminal acts. Misdirected searches merely provide a faint shadow of bliss consciousness and produce only temporary excitement and pleasure. We may try to run away from the basic puzzle of life and fear of death by covering up our actions. More covering up is done by pretending to be happy on the surface. Ultimately we become lost and confused. Yoga is a way of facing reality directly instead of running away from it. It takes a brave person to face this reality. Yoga is the path of the brave. Yoga gives direction and channels our energy so that we may find longer lasting happiness which in turn liberates us instead of binding us.

3. Yogi Patanjali defines Yoga as quieting the modifications (disturbances) of the CHITTA. Chitta is mindstuff, made of manah (mind), buddhi (intellect), and ahamkara (ego). Mind is like the surface of a lake. When this surface is disturbed by waves and impurities, the bottom cannot be seen. When chitta is freed from five kinds of disturbances (explained in detail under Raja Yoga), pure consciousness reveals itself like the bottom of the lake.

The universe that we see is a projection of our own mind. Mind is like our sunglasses. The color of the glasses distorts the true color of the objects we see. Pleasant and unpleasant experiences are produced by our state of mind. Pleasure and pain are hidden in each other. The experience of one polarizes the other. This is duality. Mind is the cause of this duality. When the mind is purified, the whole universe is perceived in its true essence, which is harmonious all the time. Duality disappears and unity in the multiplicity of the universe is experienced by the purified mind. Behind all the ornaments of gold, the essence is gold. In the same way, the essence of all existence is God (pure consciousness) although names and forms differ.

Raja Yoga techniques involve knowing the self in a systematic manner. We start with the body, nerves, and mind, and then transcend the mind. Our body is like a light bulb. The nerves are the wires, prana is the electricity. Mind is the light switch, intellect the circuit breaker. Atman is the real source of all (the Dynamo). We begin with the body and gradually reach the Atman, the real essence of our existence, and experience the highest freedom.

4. An Upanishad explains the goal of Yoga by an appropriate analogy. Our body is a chariot, the five senses are the horses, our vital energics the wheels, virtue and vice are the spokes, mind is the reins, intellect the charioteer, and Atman is the master. Life is the road on which we travel and Self-realization is our goal. We meet six enemies along the road: sensual thirst, anger, greed, pride, delusion, and hatred. The master has to awaken and bring the horses and chariot under control. With the sword of discrimination he must conquer all enemies to reach the destiny of Self-realization. The master must utilize all the instruments to reach the goal.

The Meaning and Goal of Yoga

The practice of Yoga starts with our own self. When we find the center within, harmony flows out in a natural way. This harmony is independent of external situations. When we rely on external sources for happiness, our energy becomes scattered. Life becomes like a boat that is pushed around by the waves, currents, and weather conditions. Practicing Yoga is like installing an engine in our boat so that we become master of ourselves and of our destiny.

ORIGIN OF YOGA

Yoga techniques were discovered by seers in India. They were searching for the mystery of life and ways to find everlasting happiness. They were searching for freedom from time and space, and used their bodies and minds as laboratories for experiments. As they experienced the ultimate truth, they transferred the techniques to their disciples by word of mouth. Ultimately Yogi Patanjali compiled this knowledge in the form of sutras (aphorisms) around 200 B.C.

Yoga is one of six orthodox systems of Indian philosophy. Yogi Patanjali is the father of Raja Yoga. His textbook was expounded by the yogis of later times.

YOGA IS A SCIENCE AND AN ART FOR LIVING

Yoga is a dynamic science of human existence at all levels. It is an art of harmonious living. Although it is not a religion, some branches of Yoga resemble ritualistic religious approaches.

The goal of Yoga parallels the world religions but differs from them due to its scientific approach. It is a science based upon personal experience and does not believe in blind faith or dogmas. Yoga does not interfere with any religion or belief. It encompasses all the vital religions of the world and provides personal experiences which strengthen one's personal faith.

MANY PATHS OF YOGA

There are many branches of Yoga leading to the ultimate goal of Self-realization. The choice of path or combinations of paths depends on individual temperaments and tendencies. There are four major branches of Yoga:

1. KARMA YOGA (Yoga of action)   This involves performing one's duties as a service to God without attachments to the consequences, an ideal approach for active and service-oriented persons.

2. GNANA YOGA (Yoga of knowledge or wisdom) This involves discrimination between real and unreal, using an intellectual approach and analytical techniques. This path is ideal for people with intellectual tendencies.

3. BHAKTI YOGA (Yoga of love and devotion) This approach directs love away from material things towards God and expands into love for the creation of God. It is a good approach for people with emotional tendencies.

4. RAJA YOGA (King of Yoga)   This is the most scientific Yoga. It controls the body, nerves, and mind through physical and mental disciplines.

There are several minor Yogas which can be placed under the above categories. Mantra Yoga is a Yoga of sacred invocations and sound vibrations. It is a part of Bhakti Yoga. Kundalini Yoga involves awakening the hidden energy by using many physical means and breathing techniques. Kriya Yoga also awakens energy by physical and mental means. Hatha Yoga involves physical positions and breathing techniques.

Consider the world as a school to learn spiritual lessons. All souls are in different grades and at different levels of evolution. Accept them and love them. Do not impose your ideas and models on others.

Simplify life. A simpler life gives greater joy. If you have only two dresses it becomes an easy choice as to what to wear. If you have many dresses it becomes confusing. The simpler life provides greater joy than a complex life.

2

HISTORY AND EVOLUTION OF YOGA

Yoga is an ancient science of India which has developed in stages during the last 6,000 years. It is important to know the historical development of Hinduism (Yoga is a part of Hinduism) in order to understand Yoga in its proper perspective. Hinduism includes all the religions and philosophies that have evolved in India.

The word Hindu is derived from the river Sindhu (Indus). The residents of the Sindhu River were called Hindus. Their civilization was called, "The Indus Valley Civilization," which is about 4,500 years old.

Around 2,000 B.C. the Aryan race from Central Asia invaded India and established their culture and civilization. They spoke Sanskrit and their literature was called, "The VEDAS." VEDAS are ancient literary documents of the Indo-European world and are accepted as the authoritative scriptures of the Hindus.

The word Veda is derived from the Sanskrit root Vid (to know). Veda means knowledge or wisdom. There are four Vedas: 1. Rig Veda - This contains hymns and prayers to praise various gods like sun, earth, water, fire, etc. 2. Yajur Veda - This contains the sacrificial formulas. 3. Sama Veda - This contains the melodies, and 4. Atharva Veda - This deals with magical formulas.

Each of the Vedas contains four sections:

1. Samhita - Contains the hymns and prayer mantras to please gods.

2. Brahmana - Contains rituals and sacrificial duties of the householder.

3. Aranyaka - Contains duties and meditations for the retired forest-dwellers.

4. Upanishads - Contain the philosophies and the meditations of the seers.

Vedas and Upanishads are called SRUTI (revealed scriptures), which are the authoritative textbooks. The literature of the later date is called SMRITI (remembered scriptures), which form the traditional textbooks.

Between 600 B.C. and 200 A.D. two hundred Upanishads were written. Only ten of them are the major Upanishads. These sacred scriptures contain the most vital philosophies of the Vedas, which influenced Hinduism and Yoga at a later date. Upanishads are also referred to as Vedanta because they are the concluding parts of the Vedas. (Veda + Anta = Vedanta. Anta means the end.) The literal meaning of the Upanishad is to sit at the feet of a master to receive knowledge. (upa = near, ni = down, and sad = to sit.) The authors of the Upanishads are unknown as they had no materialistic interest in preserving their names. Their wisdom and spiritual experiences are revealed in the form of parables and stories.

Upanishads disregard the ceremonial and sacrificial aspects of the Vedas and teach the direct wisdom that "Thou art That." Each individual self is potentially divine and is identical to the cosmic Self (Brahman). Their approach is non-dualistic, and they believed in Nirguna Brahman (Impersonal God without qualities).

Around 600 B.C. to 500 B.C. the great epics of Ramayana and Mahabharata were composed. Ramayana and Mahabharata are stories about Rama and Krishna respectively. Rama and Krishna lived more than 6000 years ago and both are regarded as incarnations of the Godhead.

Maha means "the great" and Bharata means "the residents of Bharata " (India). Mahabharata is the great story of the wars of the Bharatas. Krishna is the hero who took human birth to transform the world by his divine glories or LILAS (Lilas are the divine plays of Krishna, which are described in the Bhagavatam). Mahabharata teaches personal and social ethics in story form written as epic poems. Ramayana was written by sage Valmiki. Rama is the hero and an ideal human being. Many moral codes and practices are taught through the Ramayana.

Bhagavad Gita was written by sage Vyasa. It is a religious classical book written in the form of celestial songs and has a universal message for people of all ages and temperaments. Its teachings are timeless. Gita is a small part of the story of Mahabharata and is written in the form of conversations between Krishna (Lord) and Arjuna (a warrior and a devotee of Krishna). Arjuna is confused on the battlefield. Krishna clears his confusion by teaching him the philosophies of Gnana, Karma, Bhakti, and Raja Yoga. The message applies to all readers.

Life is a battlefield and the individual soul (Jiva) is confused as Arjuna is confused. Krishna is the inner-consciousness that guides the soul when it seeks sincerely. Gita contains the comprehensive synthesis of vedic sacrifices, non-dualistic Brahman, the dualism of Samkhya, and the four major branches of Yoga.

Around 300 B.C. Manusmriti was written by Manu, and Artha Shastra was written by Kautilya. Manusmriti (Dharma Shastra) describes the moral conduct (Dharma) for all members of the society. It also discusses religion and ethics. Artha Shastras describe the political and economic systems. It also deals with the military, currency, and the commercial aspects of the society.

Around 600 to 500 B.C. Jainism and Buddhism came into existence. Mahavir established Jainism and Gautama Buddha established Buddhism. Jainism and Buddhism were revolutions against the corruption in Hinduism. They revolted against the rigid ritualistic approaches and revised the understandings of the Upanishads. Both religions believe in Karma (The Law of Causation) and emphasize non-violence and compassion. Buddha is recognized as one of the greatest Yogis, and some authorities consider him as one of the incarnations of the Godhead.

Buddhism spread to China, Japan, and Southeast Asia. Bodhirama, a patriarch, took Buddha's teachings from India to China in 520 A.D. and it became Chen. When the teachings traveled from China to Japan it was called Zen, and eventually Zen Buddhism came into existence. (Chen or Zen means Dhyana or meditation.) Zen believes in sudden awakening and enlightenment.

About 2000 years ago several schools of thought systematized their philosophy and composed SUTRAS (aphorisms) to explain them. The work was done by yogis and seers who used their intuition and personal experiences instead of logical arguments. Sutras are extremely short aphorisms which contain essential meanings and cannot be understood without the commentaries. Six basic orthodox schools of thought were formed during this era. They were: 1. Nyaya 2. Vaisheshika 3. Samkhya 4. Yoga 5. Poorva Mimamsa 6. Uttar Mimamsa.

1. NYAYA This deals with logical methods of attaining knowledge. It was written in the year 300 B.C. by Gautama. Nyaya means justice or the science of right (just) understanding.

2. VAISHESHIKA This was written in 300 B.C. by Kasyapa. Vishesha means particular or individual. This gives importance to the individual personality. It is a system of physics and metaphysics dealing with the nature and creation of the universe.

3. SAMKHYA Samkhya was written in 300 A.D. by the legendary Kapila in the form of Samkhya Karika. Samkhya is known for the theory of evolution of the universe. Brahman is the all pervading reality which is one without a second.

Its two facets are Purusha and Prakriti. Purusha is the conscious principle which is the subject; Prakriti (nature or matter) is the unconscious principle, which is the object. Prakriti has three gunas (attributes or qualities), Satva, Rajas, and Tamas. SATVA (purity) or potential consciousness, RAJAS or activity, and TAMAS or inertia.

When the gunas are in equilibrium, the universe remains in unmanifest (seed) form. When Purusha excites Prakriti, the equilibrium is disturbed and Mahat, or Cosmic Intelligence, is formed. From Mahat comes Buddhi (individual intelligence). From Buddhi comes Ahamkara (ego). From Ahamkara, Satva forms Mind (manas) and five organs of action (hands, feet, speech, excretion, reproduction), and five organs of perception (hearing, smelling, tasting, touching, seeing).

From Ahamkara, Tamas forms five Tanmatras (subtle elements). These elements are earth, water, fire, air, and ether. From these Tanmatras the gross body is made. The Rajas provides energy for both Satva and Tamas.

Skillful action is Yoga. Performing activities with efficiency, love, and freedom from anxiety is Yoga.

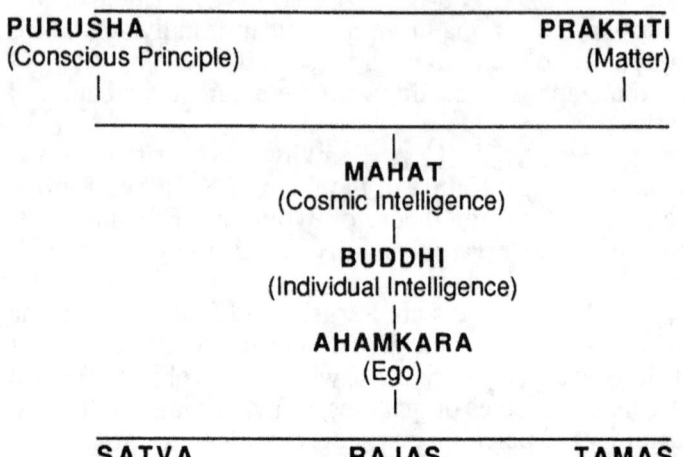

BRAHMAN
(Absolute Reality)

PURUSHA	PRAKRITI
(Conscious Principle)	(Matter)

MAHAT
(Cosmic Intelligence)

BUDDHI
(Individual Intelligence)

AHAMKARA
(Ego)

SATVA	RAJAS	TAMAS
Mind & organs of action and perception	Generates Energy for Satva and Tamas	Tanmatras (earth, water, fire, air, ether)

Manifestation of Prakriti is called evolution. Prakriti returning to seed form is called involution. Evolution and involution form a complete cycle. Purusha is always free and bondage is due to ignorance. Obstacles are removed from the path of Purusha with the practice of Yoga techniques. Moksha (liberation) is the goal of life.

4. YOGA Two hundred B.C. Yogi Patanjali wrote the textbook of Raja Yoga called <u>Yoga Sutras</u>. Raja Yoga has eight steps: Yama, Niyama, Asana, Pranayama, Pratyahara, Dharana, Dhyana, and Samadhi. These Sutras contain the techniques of physical and mental control to attain complete mastery of the mind, and they describe the theory and practice of Yoga. They also describe obstacles on the path of Yoga, supernatural powers obtained through Yoga, and various samadhis.

Bhoja and Vyasa wrote the detailed commentaries on the Yoga Sutras. Patanjali did not describe details of the physical mastery of asana and pranayama. Yogi Swatmarama wrote the textbook of Hatha Yoga called <u>HATHA YOGA</u>

PRADIPIKA around 1400-1500 A.D. by compiling the techniques which were known by word of mouth. The details of Raja Yoga and Hatha Yoga are given in Chapters 3 and 4.

5. POORVA MIMAMSA Jaimini wrote Mimamsa Sutra around 400 B.C. Poorva means earlier. Poorva Mimamsa is the earlier investigations of Vedas. It accepts Vedas as scriptural authority and describes Karma Kanda aspects (dharma or duty) of individuals.

6. UTTAR MIMAMSA or VEDANTA Uttar means later. They are later investigations of Vedas. Badarayana wrote Brahman Sutras around 500 B.C. This offers religious and philosophical speculations of the Upanishads and deals with the doctrine of Brahman, so it is called Brahma Sutras. It is also called Vedanta because it deals with the final aims of the Vedas.

Shankara, Ramanuja, and Madhavacharya wrote the commentaries on Brahma Sutras at a later date. Shankara wrote commentaries on the Vedanta around 800 A.D. (Upanishads, Bhagavad Gita, and Brahma Sutras are called Vedanta.) He interpreted the Vedanta from a non-dualistic point of view. Brahman is the basis and ground of all experiences. The Atman within each individual is identical with universal Brahman. When this truth is realized Moksha (liberation) is attained. Shankara is considered the authority on Vedanta. He also wrote VIVEKA-CHUDAMANI which is the textbook of Gnana Yoga.

Ramanuja wrote commentaries on Vedanta during the 11th Century A.D. His stand was qualified dualism, and he considered matter as the body of Brahman. God controls the universe and man's goal is to serve God. He emphasized devotion in contrast to Shankara's Gnana Yoga approach (Yoga of Knowledge).

Madhava wrote dualistic commentaries on the Vedanta around the 12th Century A.D. He emphasized the Bhakti Yoga (devotional) approach, stressing a personal God (Vishnu) as sustainer.

Around the 17th Century, scholars started writing commentaries on the commentaries using logic instead of intuition. They colored the philosophies according to their revolutionary ideas. The philosophies became diversified and more schools of thought and sub-branches were formed.

We each have specific individual personality traits, tendencies, and temperaments. We cannot forcefully control these traits without producing strain. We are an extrovert or an introvert, emotional or intellectual. If we understand our natural tendencies we can utilize them for growth instead of becoming disturbed by them.

**

Try for the best, prepare for the worst. Fears can be confronted by imagining the worst. Most fears are imaginary, created by a restless mind. Hiding from them only magnifies the fears.

**

Meditation is not a waste of time. It is a process of going inward and coming out with extra energy. Meditation is to draw on an inner source of energy and make it available in everyday life. To the extent the arrow is pulled away it goes forward. One extra inch of pull may result in many additional feet of travel.

**

Utilize all the facilities in life for meditation. Don't let them make you lethargic, arrogant, or egotistical. Let adversities in life become stepping stones to learn spiritual lessons. Welcome them as blessing in disguise.

**

Some horses must be whipped before they move, others will move with one crack of the whip. Some horses run while looking at the shadow of the whip before it strikes. Wise persons learn a lesson by looking around and observing the laws of nature. Others wait until they are whipped by nature before they wake up.

Some people build sandcastles on the beach and a large wave destroys them. We build castles of desires and merciless nature destroys them in a single moment.

**

Be like a bee that gathers honey from different flowers. Absorb only the pleasant and useful knowledge. Pluck the roses and leave the thorns behind.

****

PHILOSOPHY
and
PRACTICES

3. Raja Yoga

4. Hatha Yoga

5. Yoga Positions

6. Breathing

7. Relaxation

8. Kundalini Yoga

9. Concentration and Meditation

10. Bhakti Yoga

11. Mantra Yoga/Arti

12. Surrender Yoga

13. Guru

14. Initiation

15. Gnana Yoga

16. Reincarnation

17. Karma Yoga

3

RAJA YOGA

Raja means king. Raja Yoga is the Supreme Yoga or the King of Yoga. It is the most systematic and scientific Yoga for acquiring union with the Supreme. Raja Yoga has eight steps which prepare a person systematically and gradually for the ultimate goal of Yoga. These steps are: Yama, Niyama, Asana, Pranayama, Pratyahara, Dharana, Dhyana, and Samadhi. One step leads to the next higher step. The approach starts with the physical body by controlling the functions of the body and making it healthy, then transcending it by producing rhythm in the body by means of proper diet and exercises.

The senses, nerves, and nerve centers are controlled by practicing breathing and concentration techniques. Finally, the mind is controlled and transcended by practicing concentration and meditation.

This is a very sound approach as it is easier to control the gross body than to control the subtle mind. After mastering the gross body, the subtle mind is easily controlled.

Our body is like a light bulb. The nerves are the wires, prana the electricity; the mind and intellect are the switches. Atman is the powerhouse. We must start with the body to reach the powerhouse of Atman.

The techniques of Raja Yoga have been known for thousands of years. Yogi Patanjali compiled and systematized these techniques around 200 B.C. The textbook is entitled The Yoga Sutras (aphorisms) of Patanjali. The Sutras are very short. One hundred ninety-five Sutras fill up about two pages, but their contents require commentary. Most of the Sutras can be understood only when one reaches the higher stages of meditation and experiences for himself. The commentaries were written by various yogis from the 4th to the 16th Century A.D.

YAMAS AND NIYAMAS (Moral Disciplines) Yama means self-restraint and Niyama means self-discipline. Yama and Niyama together are the ten commandments of Yoga. These form the code of morality and ethics. Yama and Niyama are preliminary essentials which keep our being in harmony with the universe, and without which progress on the path is not possible. Also, they purify the consciousness so that one is prepared to handle the experiences and powers attained by the higher practices of Yoga. These codes produce emotional maturity and balance.

Powers attained through Yoga are like sharp weapons. Without emotional maturity one may misuse them and develop serious problems. The morality of Yama and Niyama is not a conventional morality. It is a very subtle one based upon the higher laws of nature and one's internal commitment. Though they may look forbidding, they produce maximum freedom. There is no freedom without discipline.

In an automobile the gas pedal is the freedom and the brakes are the discipline. Without the discipline of the brakes, speed would be destructive. Similarly, a river's banks are the disciplines of the river and maintain the river's structure. The river would be destroyed without its banks.

In following the disciplines, one must use judgment in considering time, place, and circumstances. They should not produce rigidity; they should be dynamic. The disciplines become subtler and subtler as one tries them. By holding on to one discipline at all costs, the student will be guided into another one. Practice of the disciplines will produce inner joy to the sincere aspirant. They become burdens to those who practice them without awareness and for show only.

Disciplines can be interwoven into our everyday life without making a show about it, then life becomes a storehouse of rewarding experiences. To master all disciplines initially will not be possible, but one should practice continually as he moves on to the next step of Yoga. The autobiography of Mahatma Gandhi is recommended for Yoga students to derive inspiration and understanding of Yama and Niyama.

1. YAMA (Restrictions) All humans have basic animal instincts which drain their energy. Survival, lust, and greed occupy a great deal of time and energy for the average person. Yama restricts the energy so it is available for spiritual awareness. By restricting these instincts, vital energy is generated and tranquility of mind is attained. There are five Yamas: A. Ahimsa or non-violence, B. Satya or truthfulness, C. Asteya or non-stealing, D. Brahmacharya or continence, and E. Aparigrahah or non-covetousness.

A. Ahimsa (Non-Violence) Ahimsa means non-killing and non-injury. In the broader sense it applies to the underlying unity of all lives. This unity is lost because of our violence. We should begin the practice with the gross form where one does not kill any life or hurt others for his selfish pleasure or gain. This involves not eating meat and not killing animals for sport and fun. Then we control our speech by speaking truth, and we do not hurt others by harsh, arrogant, and insulting speech.

Violence produced by thought is the subtlest form of violence and relatively the hardest to conquer. All violence is generated in thought form before it manifests itself in speech or action. Thinking of causing harm to anyone is also violence. No one may notice it, but you will be the first and inevitable victim of such violence. Imagine that you are mentally angry at someone. It will immediately disturb your physical and mental harmony by affecting your breathing, heart beat, and shocking your nerves and digestion.

Scattered thoughts, words, and deeds dissipate creative energy and produce restlessness. As one evolves, thoughts, speech, and actions become uniform. One finds peace. Integrated thoughts, speech, and actions provide creative energy. When this energy gains support from emotions by faith and love, fuel is added. Such a combination and integration of emotions and intellect can create miracles, besides providing spiritual bliss.

Inner mental violence should not be suppressed. As psychologists recommend, it should be taken out in some form of harmless expression to avoid physical and emotional problems. Yoga recommends a more positive approach: Transform and control the waves of anger by waves of love and compassion for all creatures. Yogi Patanjali says that when one is established in the practice of non-violence, all living creatures cease to feel enmity in his presence. This has been proven in the past by saints all over the world.

B. Satya (Truthfulness) Satya is truth. We should do truthful and honest activities. Not lying is the conventional practice of truth. There are subtle aspects of truth, such as, indulging in pretense, hiding, exaggeration, and gossiping. These must be avoided. Purity is obtained when one has harmony of thoughts, words, and deeds. When we try to manipulate truth to look good, to impress someone, or to avoid exposure for something we have done, we tell lies which produce more lies. This complicates the mind and produces many emotional problems.

This type of living is common in society. Certain expressions are used on certain occasions as a social rule which produce greater and greater distance in a person's thoughts, words, and deeds. Truth is God and God is within. By practicing truth, we come in closer contact with our inner self by producing clarity. Clarity and purity purify one's Buddhi (intellect) which helps the yogi make decisions on higher paths.

There is only one truth, which is absolute truth, others are relative truths which are always changing. One should be dynamic and able to change the interpretation of truth as it applies at any particular moment. Do not practice rigid truth. Do not manipulate truth or rationalize to make life easier. Spontaneous practice of truth leads to the absolute truth which is Brahman.

Yogi Patanjali explains that by being established in the practice of truth, the yogi attains the powers of materializing the fruits of good deeds without performing the deeds. By observing silence and uttering only truth, one's speech generates such power that his words become deeds right there and then.

C. Asteya (Non-Stealing) On the conventional level the average person does not steal, but on the subtler level very few people practice non-stealing. Attaining any reward in the form of material or credit without working for it, not working wholeheartedly for which one is paid, doing things behind someone's back, and dishonest conduct are all subtle forms of stealing. Many such forms of stealing are practiced by the average person out of habit. Desiring someone's property, or envying others is a subtle form of stealing. The practice of asteya will increase awareness. You will become open and fearless.

Positive practice of asteya is to consider the whole world as belonging to God, and we have no right to gain more than we deserve or to enjoy life when our neighbors are suffering. Although we have earned our possessions with hard work, we should give up ownership of excesses and share them wisely. According to Patanjali, when one masters asteya, all the wealth gets attracted to him. This is seen in cases of many evolved yogis where, although the whole world is at their disposal, they ignore it.

D. Brahmacharya (Continence) Brahma means the supreme being (God) and Charya means worship.

Brahmacharya means being attuned to God. In the conventional term brahmacharya is interpreted as continency or abstaining from the pleasure of sex. Everyone is born with this energy, and the sex drive is a fundamental pleasure drive in all beings. Knowingly or unknowingly, all our activities are centered around gratifying this desire. Controlling this sex energy is the first step in withdrawing our attention from the sensual world and transferring it to the spiritual world.

Yogis say that when one controls the sexual energy by thought, word, and deed, it gets converted into ojas in the forehead. Ojas is the highest form of refined subtle energy which gives one poise, inner tranquility, and mental energy. Geniuses have accumulated some ojas by intense concentration, without being consciously aware of it. The process of converting sex energy into ojas is the process of sublimation and not suppression. Suppression of sex energy is unhealthy and may cause physical and emotional problems.

In the wider sense brahmacharya means to attain freedom from cravings for sensual enjoyments. The yogi begins with physical renunciation of pleasures, giving up sexual intercourse, perfumes, fancy clothes, hair styles, stimulating food, and the company of distracting friends and environment. It is easy to give up physical things. This is the first step, yet the more difficult step comes when one has to give up the relish which persists internally, and which is removed only after long persistent practice and surrender to the Lord.

Without purity of food and mind, external brahmacharya is improbable. According to Yoga, youth is best for enjoying sensual pleasures and also best for Yoga practices. For the average householder moderation in sex is recommended. Even a small effort in observing this discipline becomes rewarding in the form of health, mental peace, and creative energy.

The serious practice of Yoga doesn't start until all cravings have subsided. This means a householder also has to observe full scale brahmacharya to attain intensity of his practices. Giving up pleasures does not mean running away from sensual situations but to transcend them. Whatever comes naturally one accepts and remains content, becoming free from likes and dislikes. According to Yogi Patanjali, one who is established in brahmacharya acquires spiritual energy.

E. Aparigrahah (Non-Greediness) Aparigrahah means non-greediness or non-possessiveness. We need a few things for survival, but we create necessities, comforts, luxuries, and accumulate these to impress others. The acquisition, maintenance, and guarding of these possessions takes a great deal of energy and produces heartache. We become attached to possessions and create the fear of losing them but at the time of death everything is left behind.

Aparigrahah also means not accepting favors and gifts. Acceptance of favors produces dependence on people and situations, and we become obliged to deviate from the path due to these obligations. In the positive application aparigrahah means simplifying life and not accumulating for the future. Share possessions and be free. Greediness also indicates a lack of faith in the Lord and His creation and represents an attitude of laziness. According to Yogi Patanjali, one who becomes steadfast in aparigrahah attains the knowledge of past, present, and future existences.

2. NIYAMA (Positive Disciplines) After controlling the negative forces of Yama, one becomes ready to cultivate the positive disciplines of Niyamas. There are five Niyamas.

A. Shaucha (Purity) We are created in the image of God. Our body, mind, and emotions are the vehicles through which the divine energy can manifest. The yogi must purify these vehicles. One should take care of the body as an instrument instead of a goal. Physical cleansing involves proper Satvik (pure) diet, fasting, and cleansing techniques to clean our internal organs from toxins. Six yogic cleansing techniques, diet, fasting, and postures are described under their respective titles, and details of the practices are given. Simple cleansing techniques, like taking frequent baths, are very sound as one can experience the difference when one takes a bath and puts on fresh clothes before meditation in contrast to ignoring these basic disciplines.

Mind and emotions can be purified by prayers, constant satsang, mantra chanting, and the practice of non-attachment. According to Patanjali, as a result of shaucha, one attains indifference towards the body, disgust for physical intercourse, cheerfulness of mind, power of concentration, control of passions, and fitness for the vision of the Atman.

B. Santosa (Contentment) Contentment gives one equilibrium which is a must for students of Yoga who wish to progress on the path. Contentment is the acceptance of all situations in life with a positive attitude avoiding comparisons, and accepting your own self.

Contentment is not produced out of laziness, nor is it an escape or fatalism where one gives up because of inability or weakness. On the contrary, one knows through his wisdom and experiences, the futility of certain activities and transcends them. Other activities that he performs do not disturb his equilibrium. Santosa produces inside out happiness. It produces awareness of the storehouse of happiness which is already part of his inner self.

Happiness arising from satisfying our lower desires is temporary. Desires increase while satisfying them; it's like pouring oil into the fire. Happiness produced by contentment is like an ocean. The ocean is calm inside while waves are flowing on the surface. Happiness produced from satisfying lower desires is like a river which looks calm on the surface but has a strong undercurrent. Patanjali explains that by mastery of contentment supreme happiness is attained. This supreme happiness is self-contained and does not depend upon any external environment.

C. Tapa (Austerity) Different practices are utilized to control our lower nature. Tapa in Sanskrit means to heat. By heating the ores, the pure metal is obtained. In the same way, the restless senses are purified through the heat of disciplines. Without austerity nothing can be attained. Study is the austerity of a student, and practice on the field while sacrificing all other pleasures for the accomplishment of one goal is the austerity of an athlete.

Austerity builds will power and spiritual strength. Yogis take different vows and stick to them at any cost. These vows may range from dietary disciplines to disciplines of various senses, which serve as a means to purify mind and senses.

Austerities are not meant for torture but are constructive self-chosen disciplines where one has a definite purpose and understanding in mind. For example, the disciplines of fasting and exercising can become starvation and labor, respectively, when done without proper understanding. One may practice austerities of the five senses: abstaining from seeing, hearing, smelling, tasting, and touching certain objects. The senses are purified when they are freed from attachments to their objects.

According to Patanjali, by practicing tapas one attains certain physical, mental, and psychic powers.

D. Swadhyaya (Self-Study) Swa means own, and Adhyaya means think or study. A person should study himself by introspection. Our external behavior has its roots in our deep mind. A seeker studies and analyzes his own life. Another meaning of swadhyaya is study of the scriptures. Scriptures provide theoretical knowledge and inspiration. It is recommended for a student of Yoga to read only authentic scriptures and books written by masters from their experience rather than reading mere intellectual study for showing off knowledge and intelligence. A mere intellectual approach makes a person a scholar which produces a hindrance on the path.

Read a few lines from the scriptures and reflect on them, and the deep meaning will be revealed to you. Scriptures provide higher thoughts to live by. Thoughts are very potent. They turn into words and deeds. Thoughts are like seeds which should be nurtured by constant practice so that a spiritual tree may be produced from them.

Satsang of holy saints and friends, and constant mantra chanting are good means of swadhyaya whenever the mind is idle. According to Patanjali, by practicing swadhyaya, one attains the vision of the aspect of God which is worshiped.

E. Ishwara Pranidhana (Surrender to God) Ishwara pranidhana means surrender to Ishwara (God) or resign to the will of God, uniting the limited will to that of the Supreme. The yogi accepts all seemingly pleasant and unpleasant circumstances as the will of God and saves his energy by avoiding unnecessary struggle.

Surrender is not a weakness or giving up but is a positive asset of a yogi. It is a positive affirmation of seeing the large scale potential of our existence. Surrender Yoga, Chapter 12, explains the details of this principle. By surrendering we become an instrument rather than a doer and become free from tension and karmas (impressions) produced by the feelings of doership. This doership or "I consciousness" is called Asmita which is the root cause of all kleshas (suffering).

Surrender also helps in attaining non-attachment. As described in the Gita, one should practice constant surrender. If it is hard, perform all actions to please God. If this is also hard, surrender the fruits of actions to God. This surrender of the fruits of all actions produces instant and lasting peace. By practicing Ishvara pranidhana one attains samadhi (ultimate union), which is the highest goal of Yoga.

Patanjali believes Ishwara is the Cosmic Brahman seen through the human mind. Brahman includes everything while Ishwara is a special being, a personal God, who is the ruler of the universe. He is free from karma and its effects and manifests infinite knowledge. Brahman is not limited by time and is the teacher of all ancient teachers. He is expressed through the word OM. One should meditate on the meaning of OM. It brings the knowledge of Atman which removes ignorance.

3. ASANA (Position) (See details on practical aspects of asanas in Chapter 5, Yoga Positions.) The third state of Raja Yoga is called asana or positions. Asana means placing the body in a steady and comfortable position for a prolonged period. Restlessness in the body produces restlessness in the mind. When the body is disciplined to stay in a steady position for a longer period, one is considered a master of that position. After doing the position, one is able to transcend the distraction of the body and is free to control the senses and the mind.

Yogi Patanjali refers to the positions Padmasana (lotus) and Siddhasana(Adept's Pose). Both are meditative positions where one crosses his legs and the body is in perfect balance, the chest, neck, and head are kept in a perfectly straight line. By keeping the spine in a vertical position, the nerve current can flow smoothly through the spine. This keeps the mind alert and allows progress in meditation.

The steady position is not a forced or rigid position which produces tension but is acquired by controlling the natural tendencies of the body. Consciousness is lifted from the body, and the subconscious mind maintains steadiness in the body. It is recommended to meditate on the infinite to attain steadiness of the posture. One should rise above the pairs of opposites like heat and cold, noise, and other sensations, to attain this stability.

On the other hand, when mastery is attained over the position, one is able to rise above physical sensations which are distractions in meditation. Mastery of postures brings control of the life force, and one becomes ready for the next step which is pranayama.

Yogi Patanjali's interest is in the attainment of spiritual illumination and does not describe details of the postures. Hatha Yoga describes these details. There are eighty-four major postures. They affect the internal mechanisms of the body, which control our breathing, circulation, nerves, glands, spinal cord, internal organs of digestion, metabolism, and elimination.

Practice of Yoga positions frees the body from toxins, removes blocks of tension, and increases endurance which helps maintain the meditative position for a longer time. All postures, directly or indirectly, prepare for this aim of maintaining freedom from the body.

4. PRANAYAMA (Breathing Control)
(See Chapter 6, Breathing, for the techniques of pranayama.)

Prana means the vital energy, and Ayam means control or regulation. Pranayama means the techniques of controlling the vital air (prana). The whole universe is pervaded by matter and energy. Prana is the subtlest essence of energy that exists in the universe. This energy is neither good nor bad, neither negative nor positive. It manifests in the form of heat, light, sound, mechanical energy, or mind power and exists in all living creatures. In the absence of this energy, humans are pronounced dead. With this prana we see, hear, and think. It expresses itself in different ways at different levels of consciousness. By controlling prana one can control his body, mind, and the forces of the universe.

Breathing is the flywheel of our life. This fundamental motion sets up all other motions in our body. In the gross form breathing seems to be like prana so prana is interpreted as breath, and control of breath is interpreted as pranayama.

In the higher forms, one learns to control the subtle prana which flows through pranamaya kosha or our subtle body and controls our subtle functions. Physical pranayama brings oxygenation and rejuvenation to the cells, tissues, and vital organs of the body. It provides energy to the organs of digestion, elimination, and the nervous system. Breathing and our emotional states are closely connected. By slowing down and producing the rhythm of breathing, one controls his emotional nature and becomes ready for the next step of controlling the senses. Pranayama also unites the body and mind and produces harmony between them.

Pranayama techniques involve purak or inhalation, kumbhak or retention of breath, and rechak or exhalation. The retention can be internal or external, and the practice depends upon time, place, climate, and other conditions. Basic pranayama can be practiced by an individual as described in this book, but advanced pranayama requires the guidance of an experienced teacher. The higher pranayama involves subtler control of prana; one's external breathing stops altogether.

Mastery of pranayama removes the coverings which hide the light of the mind. Rajasik and Tamasik qualities are removed. Consciousness becomes purified and qualifies one for the practice of concentration.

5. PRATYAHARA (Sense Withdrawal)

Prati means withdrawal and Ahara means food. Pratyhara means withdrawing the senses from their respective objects. Mind works through the senses. When the mind is withdrawn from sense objects, the senses also withdraw from them. When the senses are exposed to their pleasure objects, but mind is disconnected from the senses, sensations are not perceived. Pratyahara gives one mastery of the senses and the energy which was going outward through the senses is directed inward. The five senses are the gates which establish contact with the external world. When this contact is broken, we are able to travel to the kingdom of heaven within.

There is pratyahara practice for each sense. For example, pratyahara of hearing may be practiced by listening to an orchestra and concentrating on one instrument to the exclusion of all others. Also, the yogi may ignore all distracting noises and remain attuned to his activities, or he may produce desired sounds in the inner ear without actual existence of any sound. Listening to an inner OM sound is such a practice of pratyahara.

Pratyahara of sight includes seeing one object to the exclusion of all others, or focusing the closed eyes between the eyebrows and seeing the shining light. In the same way, there is pratyahara for smell, taste, and touch. Uncontrolled senses are destructive. The fish is destroyed due to the attraction to taste. A bee is destroyed due to the attraction of smell. A moth is killed due to the attraction of light. A snake is caught due to attraction to sound; and an elephant is caught due to the attraction of touch. Human beings with five strong senses must learn to control them.

6. DHARANA (Concentration) (See Chapter 9, Concentration and Meditation, for details and techniques.) Dharana means concentration, or holding the mind steady on a single object. We become worthy of concentration after mastering the previous limbs of Raja Yoga.

Yama and Niyama remove emotional disturbances, postures remove physical disturbances, pranayama removes disturbances produced by the nervous system and pratyahara removes disturbances of the senses.

Concentration on external objects is called Tratak (as in concentrating on a candle flame), which is a Hatha Yoga technique for cleansing. Conventional concentration techniques are used for material success. The purpose of concentration in Yoga is to make the mind one-pointed so that it can be focused inward to know our own self.

The power of mind is like the rays of the sun. When the dissipated rays are accumulated at one point, they generate tremendous heat. In the same way, concentration generates one-pointedness and sharpness of mind which enable one to perform many feats. Mind is the miracle house of the humans. One can uncover hidden powers through the techniques of concentration.

Yogi Patanjali recommends concentration on the chakras (subtle psychic centers within the spine). Another common practice of concentration is to focus on the agnya chakra, the center between the eyebrows, or on the tip of the nose.

7. DHYANA (Meditation) (See Chapter 9, Concentration and Meditation, for details and techniques.) Dhyana means meditation. Prolonged concentration or the unbroken flow of thoughts towards an object is called meditation. If concentration is like dripping water, meditation is like a continuous flow of water. In concentration the mind becomes one-pointed, while in meditation the mind flows harmoniously and brings wisdom and intuition. Meditation is always transcendental in nature (transcending the mind and body).

8. SAMADHI (Complete Absorption)
Sama means together and Adha means to direct. Samadhi means directing together or uniting the lower consciousness with the higher consciousness. Continuous practice of meditation leads into samadhi. In samadhi all thought forms, their meaning, and distortions and perceptions of mind disappear. Samadhi produces bliss and freedom from the dualities of the world. Higher knowledge is attained, which is beyond inference and scriptures. It wipes out past karmas and samskaras.

There are two basic stages of samadhi: sabija samadhi and nirbija samadhi. Like a crystal that takes the color of the object that is near it, so the mind attains sameness with the object of meditation. Subject and object merge, and one obtains direct knowledge.

SABIJA SAMADHI Sabija samadhi is samadhi with seed and has ego or I consciousness. There is union with God while in this state of samadhi, but in the normal state we return to the basic human tendencies. We can fall from this samadhi easily. There are various stages in sabija samadhi: 1.Reasoning, 2. Discrimination, 3. Bliss, and 4. A sense of pure consciousness.

The early stage is called savitarka and nirvitarka samadhi. In savitarka samadhi mind achieves identity with gross objects and is aware of their name, quality, and knowledge. In nirvitarka samadhi one transcends their name and quality. In savitarka and nirvitarka samadhi one functions at manomaya kosha (mind sheath).

When the mind attains identity with the subtle object and one is aware of names and forms, it is called savichara samadhi, and when one transcends the names and forms, one attains nirvichara samadhi. In savichara and nirvichara samadhi one functions at vignanamaya kosha (intellectual sheath).

The next higher state of samadhi is sananda samadhi where one functions at anandamaya kosha (bliss sheath). Then in sasmita samadhi one functions at the level of the Atman.

NIRBIJA SAMADHI In all the above stages of sabija samadhi one is still under the influence of Prakriti (nature) and its gunas, and is open to the chances of being deluded by maya (illusion) and falling from his path. A few yogis who pass through the stages of sabija samadhi attain nirbija samadhi or the samadhi without the seed of I consciousness. One becomes free from the bonds of maya and is free from the bonds of birth and death.

This is the final liberation, the ultimate goal of Yoga. After attaining this stage, the yogi merges with the forces of nature. He has no more desire to sustain the human body. Some yogis volunteer to serve the human race and sustain their body to teach. They function through the body and manifest all the human qualities, yet their consciousness is always in tune with the Supreme. They work as a master of maya and not as a slave. Their sub-conscious impressions are like burned seeds, which do not produce any effect, and their new activities do not produce any karmas.

In nirbija samadhi the object of meditation is consciousness itself. After attaining this samadhi one is no longer deluded. While one is going through the stages of sabija samadhi and lacks non-attachment and has desires, he reaps the fruits of his samadhi by getting the position of a disincarnate God. When his good karma expires, he is incarnated in the human body again and continues his quest for liberation.

Samyama When the yogi brings concentration, meditation, and samadhi to a single subject, it is called samyama. Samyama produces intuitive knowledge, wisdom, and he discovers various stages of consciousness. By practicing samyama on different subjects and objects, a yogi is able to gain various siddhis (supernatural powers). There are eight main yogic siddhis described. Yogi Patanjali names these powers and the practices to attain them in a scientific manner, yet he warns students that these powers are traps and are dangerous. When one gives up all powers, he becomes qualified to attain nirbija samadhi.

Aids to Samadhi Yogi Patanjali recommends the following disciplines for attaining success in samadhi: faith, energy, memory, concentration, and illumination. Faith has to be dynamic, non-dogmatic and scientific. It is open to question and experience. Scriptures and the teachings of the Guru are the direction for faith, and personal experience strengthens this faith. One needs energy to sustain his practices. Progress depends upon this energy and intensity. Memory is the recollection of previous experiences, which saves time and energy.

Obstacles There are nine basic obstacles in the practice of samadhi. They are: 1. Sickness, 2. Dullness, 3. Doubt, 4. Lack of enthusiasm, 5. Laziness, 6. Cravings for happiness, 7. Delusion, 8. Despair due to failure in concentration, and 9. Unsteadiness in concentration. They manifest themselves in symptoms such as grief, mental distress, unsteadiness of body, and irregular breathing.

Yogi Patanjali recommends the following remedies for them: one-pointed concentration on a single truth, friendliness, compassion, and gladness. We should be happy for the good fortune of others and non-attached to the vices of others. He also recommends concentration on breath, concentration on subtle elements, meditation on the inner light at the third eye (between the eyebrows), meditation on the heart of an illumined soul, meditation on dream experiences, or meditation on desired objects.

Yogi Patanjali defines Yoga as controlling the modifications of chitta (mind stuff). Chitta includes three faculties of the mind: 1. Manah means mind which records all experiences, 2. Buddhi is intellect, which discriminates all the experiences, and 3. Ahamkara or ego (I consciousness) identifies and establishes the subject-object relation. Ego is the stem around which intellect and mind function. Without ego there is no mind. From this ego spring all desires, emotions, and mental disturbances.

In the background of ego exists our pure Self(Atman), which is free. It is omnipresent, omnipotent, and omniscient. Atman is pure and exists within each individual but is hidden by the mental waves, as the bottom of a lake is hidden by surface agitations and waves. When the mental agitations are removed, Atman is experienced. Experiencing Atman which brings liberation is the goal of Yoga.

There are five kinds of mental disturbances:

1. **PRAMANA** Direct perception. Perceptions which are perceived directly or indirectly and provide proof of their existence. Pratyaksha is the direct experience seen with one's own eyes or heard with one's own ears. You see the sun and know it, and are convinced about it without any doubt. Anumana is inference, or the assumption based on clues. There is smoke, and you know fire exists because of inference.

Agama is scriptural testimony, or predictions based upon direct experience. Scriptures are the direct revelation of the seers. We can also predict certain situations because of previous experiences. For example, we can predict that there will be steam when water is put on fire.

2. **VIPARYAYA** Wrong or distorted knowledge. Any knowledge which is perceived directly or indirectly, which is not true because of certain factors, is called viparyaya. In the darkness one sees a rope and believes it to be a snake. When the lights are turned on the snake disappears and the rope remains.

3. **VIKALPA** Vikalpa is delusion or hallucination. The image is produced by a word with no substance behind it. Mirage and daydreaming are examples of this. The same word may produce different images in different people depending upon their association.

4. NIDRA Nidra means sleep with or without dreams. In dreamless sleep there is an absence of any content in the mind. Here the mental waves and disturbances exist but contact with the mind and brain is broken so one does not seem to perceive any experience. It is like a car in neutral which does not move, yet the engine is running. In the same way, in deep slumber mental waves exist but are not registered. When one wakes up he remembers only that he had a nice sleep. The inner consciousness witnesses the sleep state.

5. SMRITI Memory. Memory is the recall of all previous experiences. The above four modifications can be recalled from their place of hiding within our subconscious mind. Dreams are recalls of such experiences. We can also recall previous experiences by conscious effort.

When one removes all modifications of the mind, he establishes himself in his own nature which is pure Self (Atman). This is possible in the state of samadhi. At all other times one identifies with the experience of chitta, which is constantly changing.

Yogi Patanjali recommends two fundamental methods in combination to gain mastery of the mental waves and attain freedom. They are: ABHYASA or constant practice, and VAIRAGYA or non-attachment. Practice and non-attachment should be done simultaneously. Practice without non-attachment is not possible, and if one tries he will be miserable following rigid practices as a torture. Non-attachment without practice will become fatalistic, and one will become lazy and have no direction to follow.

ABHYASA Persistent practice which leads to mastery of mental modifications is called abhyasa. This practice may involve any step of Raja Yoga for which one is ready. One must take a step forward from where he stands. Abhyasa becomes firmly established when practice is continued for a long time without interruption and with hearty love for it. Most people who desire to grow on the path of Yoga don't seem to make progress because they do not keep up with their path long enough for it to bear fruits. They dig too many shallow holes at various places and do not find water. This is due to their attachment to results. If results do not come quickly, they take another path and will surely change paths again and again.

Almost everyone knows what the good things are that they can do. If they take just one thing at a time and work on it persistently, they will find enough guidance from within.

Many persons try to follow several difficult disciplines which are intellectually appealing to them. They don't succeed in mastering them, and they become frustrated and feel guilty. Many people continually shop for a right Guru or a right path, and waste time in intellectual pursuits.

Abhyasa may also include all related activities which will help those on the path by providing inspiration. Practice is the main goal and all activities which are done to aid in this pursuit are also abhyasa. Without non-attachment one does not develop enough patience to keep up the commitment to the practices.

VAIRAGYA Non-attachment/Renunciation (For details, see Meditation Manual.) Vairagya means renunciation or non-attachment, or more specifically, giving up the cravings of the mind for objects seen and unseen. Everyone has a thirst for pleasure and enjoyment. Vairagya means freedom from Raga and Dwesha. Raga means strong attraction and Dwesha means strong repulsion. These forces produce strong likes and dislikes to materials, people, and situations in life. These forces are hidden within and oppose each other, producing the dualities of life.

A strong like for something will produce a dislike for its opposite. If one has a strong desire for receiving honor, he will be equally afraid of insult. This attraction and repulsion produces great disturbance in the mind, and freedom from them brings inner peace.

Process of Attachment Attachments come from association. If you are surrounded by people who have certain clothes, car, or furniture, or if you see a commercial on TV, it makes an impression on the mind. If the mind entertains the thought for a while, it creates a desire for attaining that object. It takes a great deal of our energy to attain it.

Desires can never be satisfied. Continually fulfilling desires is like pouring kerosene into a fire. Desires increase and turn into cravings. Cravings produce restlessness and disturb our peace. By fulfilling desires repeatedly, one forms habits, and habits build character. Any desire which is not fulfilled creates anger in the mind. Anger produces infatuation, loss of memory, and loss of discrimination. One forgets his goal of life and takes the wrong direction.

Material Attachments The aspirant should start the practice of non-attachment with material possessions. Simplify life and possess only those things which are useful instead of good looking. Enjoy the materials as if they are borrowed and can be snatched away at any moment. With this awareness you will not be possessed by possessions. You will derive good use of material things instead of just collecting them. For example, a library book which is borrowed is read quickly, while a purchased book will collect dust on the shelf.

Maintain an awareness that material things are only a means. For example, a car is a means of transportation. If you identify yourself with your new car, a scratch on the car will hurt as if you got scratched yourself. There is no harm in possessions, only the attachment to them. One can be non-attached to his palace and be happy, while another can be attached to his hut and be unhappy. Possess fewer material objects, those which are necessary and practical. Take care of them but do not become possessed by them. If you become possessed, damage or loss of them will disturb your peace. If desires exceed one's material status, one becomes unhappy. When desires are reduced, one finds contentment. Give up all desires and expectations in life, and you will find instantaneous happiness.

Start with the practice of abstinence from enjoyment of material objects. Even after giving up physical objects, our mind takes delight in thinking about them. This relish persists for a very long time and is a subconscious attachment which is hard to conquer. This disappears after the experience of Atman within. The sweetness of bread disappears after tasting honey. After experiencing the joy of Atman, attraction for other attachments fades away.

Attachment to Body We have a tendency to identify ourselves with our body. If it is beautiful, healthy, and in good shape, it makes us happy. If it is ugly, too fat, too thin, unhealthy, we are unhappy. The body is always subject to change. It can gain or lose weight and will go through sickness, disease, old age, and death. If we find freedom from attachment to the body, we can use it fully as a temple of God for Self-realization. We should spend more time in maintenance of our body than maintenance of our house, car, or furniture. We should not spend excessive time in decorating or pampering the body.

Attachment to Ideas If we are attached to certain ideas and beliefs, it will hurt us when we face others with different ideas, beliefs, and religions. It will make our minds and hearts narrow and will hinder the spiritual learning process.

Letting go of such attachments will allow us to love others and have compassion for others.

We should let go of the attachment of trying to impress others. It drains a lot of energy maintaining a certain image in society to please our friends and relatives. We should be ourselves and please the Lord within.

Attachment to Habits Any activity done for some time becomes an unconscious act which is a habit. Bad habits, such as smoking, drinking, drugs, etc., make us dependent on them for our happiness while causing damage to our body, nerves, and mind. Habits can be removed by the reverse process. Do the activity with greater awareness, and you will be free from the addiction.

Build some positive habits to rise above negative habits. Ultimately, one rises above all habits and learns to live in the present and to enjoy life spontaneously.

Emotional Attachments Emotional attachments are harder to master. Love for our family members and friends becomes attachment. We love them so much that we want to possess them. We worry about them, impose our desires and ideals on them, and have expectations of them. Many times love creates jealousy and fear of loss. If we learn to love them unconditionally as they are, with no strings attached, it will bring closeness and sweetness in the family. When you stop imposing your ideas on your loved ones, they will listen to you. Attachment produces a barrier in the flow of love.

Non-attachment to family does not mean giving up loving them, nor caring for them, nor being indifferent. When you love family and friends with attachment, you expect something from them. You want them to be happy and to possess them. This interferes with true love and produces misery. A surgeon is not able to operate on his wife due to attachment.

If one tries to help someone and is affected by the success or failure produced by this service, he is not able to perform his work without distractions. If you volunteer to work in a nursing home and deal with patients with varieties of ailments, you will feel drained of your energy if you are attached, and will feel rejuvenated if you are not attached. Non-attachment gives us the freedom of loving our family and friends as they are. Emotional attachments produce pleasure and pain, happiness and unhappiness, excitement and depression, while non-attachment produces evenness of mind and mastery of emotions.

Raja Yoga

Non-attachment is a positive attitude allowing the desired direction of energy without being influenced by emotions. When there is no desire or expectation there is peace.

We should remember that life is a journey and we are the travelers. When we travel on vacation and meet many other travelers, we enjoy their company but do not get attached to them. We stay in a motel for the night and don't get attached to the comfort or discomfort of the bed, furniture, color of the room, curtains, or available services. Such an attitude towards the journey of life prevents us from attachments. It also protects us from hurts and disappointments.

We see changes all around us: in the universe, with the seasons, day and night, pleasure and pain, changes in the human body from youth, maturity, old age, and death.

The attainment of wealth, pleasure, fame, and power is changing constantly. A person can be very famous one day and forgotten a week later. Wealth can come and be lost very quickly.

If we remember the transient nature of the universe and everything in it, we can free ourselves from attachments and enjoy living in the present moment.

If we can remain aware that life is a stage and we are the actors, then we can play our role without losing awareness of our true identity. In this way, we can enjoy life (enjoy our part in the play), without becoming attached to our role and without taking it too seriously.

<u>Attachment to Ego</u> This is the highest kind of renunciation. All attachments hang onto the concept of I and Mine. As we let go of our ego, we expand our consciousness and feel contentment in all situations. Like leaves falling off the trees in the fall, attachments drop off naturally without effort when one rises above ego.

The highest kind of non-attachment comes with giving up the thirst for life itself. When the fear of death is conquered, there are no more fears. The futility of attachment is seen. The body inevitably becomes old, suffers, and dies. Since the world is only transitory, why chase it like a mirage? This non-attachment comes from inner wisdom and is lasting. Most people get smashana vairagya from time to time (cemetery non-attachment). A person becomes non-attached to the world when he sees others dying or suffering, but this fades away as soon as other objects of pleasure are found.

Non-attachment is not becoming a fatalist. A fatalist is not interested in work. He does not perform work out of fear, but is always interested in results. A yogi works wholeheartedly with no thought of results, and gives up any desires for the fruits. By giving up desires for the fruits of labor, we give up all anxieties, put all our efforts into work, and attain success and mental peace. If there is excitement or worry about the future, progress will be hindered.

Practice of non-attachment should be mental. One should withdraw his mind from the thirst for pleasure while physically restraining his senses. Controlling the senses with sheer force while the mind is dwelling on pleasure is like controlling wild horses with reins. Wild horses can be tamed, but if they are controlled with force, they will take revenge.

We should tame our mind. Forceful disciplines will push mind, body, and senses into action with great intensity. Non-attachment should be practiced with such an understanding that one does everything without being affected by anything. A lotus leaf lives in water, yet water does not touch it. A yogi remains in the world, yet he rises above it.

Attachments obstruct the experience of love, producing feelings of ownership and possession. It leads to jealousy and fear of loss. How can a person truly love when his mind is occupied by these distractions? Attachment makes one aware of his limited self, and he feels separated from the rest of the world. Non-attachment allows one to lose himself and expand his awareness. Attachment produces selfishness and bondage while non-attachment brings selflessness and freedom. Non-attachment brings peace of mind.

Non-attachment means remaining adaptable and flexible with situations. In a severe storm rigid, large, and strong trees are chopped up by the wind, while flexible trees bend with the wind and are unharmed when the storm passes.

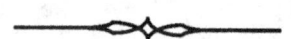

4

HATHA YOGA

As was explained in the chapter on Raja Yoga, there are eight steps to the perfection of Raja Yoga. The first four deal with the body and physical disciplines, making up what is known as Hatha Yoga. Hatha Yoga prepares one with the physical disciplines needed to master the last four stages of Raja Yoga. The steps involved in Hatha Yoga are Yama and Niyama (moral disciplines), Asana (positions), and Pranayama (control of breath). The word Ha stands for sun, and the word Tha stands for moon. Hatha Yoga means solar and lunar Yoga. The human body contains solar (positive) and lunar (negative) currents. Hatha Yoga establishes equilibrium of positive and negative currents which is needed to keep the body in a healthy condition.

Hatha Yoga is a necessary tool to master Raja Yoga. It is hard for anyone to control the mind without control of the body. The purpose of Hatha Yoga is to keep the body in a healthy and fit condition in order to withstand the hardships of the higher practices of Yoga. Yoga positions remove impurities and help the student master pranayama. Mastery of pranayama is not possible without purifying the body. Postures produce harmony within the body so that one becomes free from physical disturbances.

It is possible for a very few strong willed persons to bypass Hatha Yoga and master Raja Yoga. Some people who earned the physical mastery in their last incarnation may be able to practice and master meditation with no physical disciplines. On the other hand, one may practice Hatha Yoga and attain perfect mastery of the body, control of all the involuntary organs, prolong his life span, and remain youthful; yet it serves no purpose if one does not utilize his healthy body as an instrument to master his mind and attain liberation.

Our body is like a boat. We should utilize the boat for crossing the ocean of sansara (world of suffering) while taking good care of the boat. If we take care of the boat and do not use it, it will not take us anywhere.

Hatha Yoga, by itself, improves health but does not promise any miracles. It is a pure physical science. If, for example, one has inherited poor health, or begins Yoga practice at an advanced age, it may require more time and effort to acquire perfect health. It is never too late to start Yoga practice as no effort will be wasted.

Hatha Yoga has been known for thousands of years. In the past there was more interest in direct meditation. There was no detailed textbook written on Hatha Yoga. Sometime between 1300 to 1600 A.D. Yogi Swatmarama wrote the textbook of Hatha Yoga called Hatha Yoga Pradipika. Other textbooks of Yoga include Gheranda Samhita, Shiva Samhita, and Goraksha Paddhati.

ASANA

Asana means seat or a steady position. Yogi Patanjali defined Asana to be a firm and steady position for meditation (e.g., Lotus posture). It is not easy for the average person to maintain a single steady position for a long period of time because of toxins in the body, tensions, and pains which produce distractions. When the body is purified with various positions, diet, and cleansing techniques, one masters the steady, meditative position. The body is the vehicle for the soul. We must take good care of it for the purpose of providing a clean temple for the God (Atman) within.

We have to deal with the body constantly in our everyday life and cannot disregard it when practicing mental or spiritual disciplines. Most religions of the world emphasize moral and spiritual disciplines without emphasizing physical disciplines.

The practice of Yoga positions produces steadiness of the body and mind, agility, balance, endurance, vitality, and perfect health. One may be perfectly healthy and not strong, while a very strong person may not be healthy. A healthy person has harmony of body and mind; the body is free from all impurities, and one has peace of mind.

HOW SHOULD ONE PRACTICE YOGA POSITIONS?

Yoga postures are unique in their effects on the body and mind. For the benefits to be derived, they must be done properly. How you do the postures is very important. Positions are done differently than gymnastics, aerobics, or popular exercises. The beginner may need to spend lots of time in the earlier stages to break wrong habits in doing the exercises. The following suggestions will be helpful for Yoga students:

Yoga postures are done very gently. We want to work with our body as a friend rather than fighting it. By studying our body we gradually master it and produce harmony within. There is no comparison or competition with anyone. Every person is an individual and has to grow and progress at his own rate. One does not push nor overextend himself, so at the end he is not tired. Popular exercises make a person tired, while Yoga rejuvenates immediately, and the effect lingers on the rest of the day.

Postures are done in such a gentle way that persons of all ages can do them. Even handicapped and sick people can do many of them as taught by an experienced teacher. Persons who are bedridden can do certain simple stretches, breathing exercises, and mental control practices to improve their condition. Postures are more than exercises. They are more than a half hour to a one hour routine every day. They become part of our life by increasing our awareness during the day. Hatha Yoga makes you aware of your posture while walking, sitting, or working, and in each movement made during the day. Also, it makes you aware of your breathing, mental attitude, speech, and actions. As we become more aware of our self, we master our body and mind.

Unlike other exercises, Yoga does not work only on the body but on the body and mind simultaneously. Yoga recognizes body and mind to be an integral part of each other. Mind is the subtle part while body is the grosser part. They affect each other. Mind is the cause and body is the effect (symptom). Since body is the symptom and mind the cause, one must take care of the cause for permanent healing of the symptom. Researchers have proven that most of our physical problems begin in the mind. By working simultaneously, one obtains complete harmony of body and mind.

Most physical exercises emphasize certain areas of the body for tone, looks, or muscle development, while neglecting other areas of the body. Yoga considers our body to be a complete and wholesome unit. All areas are interconnected and affect each other. Yoga has exercises for the neck, eyes, organs, muscles, joints, and glands - for the entire body.

Yoga emphasizes the internal vital organs of circulation, respiration, digestion, elimination of impurities, the spine, nervous system, and endocrine glands, along with taking care of the muscles and joints. Vital organs control our health, determine our longevity, and remove diseases and infection-producing toxins. Other exercises overwork the muscles in building and shaping them but in later age, when the muscles are not used properly, they make a person heavy with fat. Overworking the muscles also produces exertion and strain which accelerates the aging process.

All the movements in postures are done slowly. Slow motion allows us to be aware of our body in contrast to a mechanical workout. New things are discovered about our body and its functioning. This awareness is the first step towards mastery of our body and the ability to heal it ourselves. Slow motion brings harmony between body and mind. This becomes a form of meditation. Meditation which involves body movements of this kind is an easier meditation for beginners.

Physically, this type of slow motion provides a better stretch to the deeper muscles of the body than the faster exercises. One can tone up his or her body only by affecting deep muscles. Also, the muscles are stretched and lengthened in Yoga instead of shrinking. Muscles are toned by stretching them in this fashion. One gets enough exercise by doing the movements slowly, and doing each posture only one or twice.

Postures are positions. The important aspect of postures is to get into the position and maintain it for a longer time. Certain specific benefits are derived by holding that particular position, which cannot be obtained simply by rapid or acrobatic movements.

Each posture is done with full concentration. Keeping the eyes closed while doing them is recommended. Do not do Yoga while watching TV, talking to someone, or thinking extraneous thoughts. Maintain the position and remain aware of the benefits being derived from that posture. Talk to the inner organs, communicate with them, and establish a biofeedback response. Also, concentrate on slow movements.

Each movement should be coordinated with the breathing. Retention of postures involves retention of breath, held in or held out, depending upon the position. Breathing nourishes the cells of the body while exercising them. This rejuvenates the body instead of tiring it. In heavy exercises one runs out of breath (as in jogging), and feels oxygen starvation. Breath is the link between the body and mind. One finds harmony and integration of body and mind by coordinating his breathing. Breathing also helps in getting a better stretch, better coordination, and balance. Breathing increases the lung capacity and gives better circulation to areas which are affected by those positions.

Each posture is ended with relaxation on the back and with deep breathing. Deep relaxation allows the body to rest and normalize the inner organs which were exercised by the posture.

GENERAL RULES AND PREPARATION FOR HATHA YOGA

Set aside time for practice of Yoga in the morning and in the evening. If this is not possible, practice at least one time during the day. Use the same time and place to derive optimum benefits. There should be no distractions, mental worry, or rush of any kind at that time.

Take a shower or bath and put on fresh clothes. Stomach, bladder, and bowels should be empty. Clothes should be loose and comfortable. Use a good carpet and open some windows to ventilate the room.

Do each posture very gently with coordinated breathing and concentration. Practice within your capacity without rush or push. For mastering difficult postures, mentally visualize yourself doing those postures, and they will come to you easily. Concentrate on the benefits as you retain the position. Relax for a short time after each position and take a longer rest at the end of the routine.

Be regular and moderate in eating and sleeping. Eat yogic meals, avoid over-eating, fast once a week, and avoid alcohol, meat, and stimulants for progress in Yoga practice. Keep the company of friends who inspire you on the higher path and read inspirational books. Avoid unnecessary disturbing activities.

GENERAL BENEFITS OF YOGA

Yoga is a wholesome science of body, mind, and spirit. It provides many benefits. Each and every person can use Yoga because the benefits that it offers are of a wide range. If one spends about half an hour daily in the practice of Yoga, he will receive benefits which will save him time, energy, and doctor bills; it will also provide him with a better physical and mental disposition. One will not need as much sleep or food and can work for more hours without getting tired. One will feel better, enjoy life, and accept all situations in life. These changes are real and can be verified by a doctor's check-up, or will soon be noticed by your friends and yourself.

Yoga is a preventive science, preventing problems before they arise. It keeps the body in rhythm and harmony, and removes toxins which cause problems. However, it is equally ideal for cures of many problems and diseases. Many so-called incurable diseases can be cured by Yoga practice, proper yogic diet, fasting, and meditation. The teacher of Yoga must have the knowledge and experience to help the students. Most cures take a longer time. It is not an instant method of taking medicine and curing the symptoms or hiding the problem, but it removes the root causes of problems. Patience and faith are required. However, the following basic day-to-day problems and diseases can be avoided or cured without elaborate disciplines.

Tension Tension is the root cause of our basic problems. The nervous system controls most of the physiological functions of the body. Just by learning to relax properly one can eliminate basic health problems. Yoga offers breathing techniques which are very helpful for general relaxation, insomnia, and for controlling emotional disturbances. Rhythmic breathing is ideal for insomnia. Neck exercises remove basic tension headaches. Headstand and shoulderstand are ideal for removing general problems of tension.

Cleansing Nature has devised four basic organs in our body to remove accumulated toxins. They are: kidneys, lungs, skin, and large intestine. These organs will become clogged from time to time when they are overused or abused. Yoga has six basic cleansing techniques which remove toxins from the body (described in Chapter 23, Cleansing). Most of the positions have some effect on these basic functions to help keep the body clean.

Endocrine Glands Endocrine glands are ductless glands. They secrete their hormones directly into the blood stream. These glands control most of the functions of our body and establish the body's chemical balance. The basic endocrine glands are: pituitary, pineal, thyroid, parathyroid, adrenals, pancreas, ovaries, and testes. The circulation provides raw material to the glands from which they form final chemical substances called hormones. Hormones circulate through the body and affect various functions. Endocrine glands also control other organs and their functions. The headstand and shoulderstand affect most of the endocrine glands, while other postures affect some of them.

Involuntary Organs Most of the positions control the involuntary organs and establish the rhythm of their functions. They influence digestion by affecting the stomach, digestive glands, and their secretions. They stimulate the organs of elimination and help remove waste from the larger intestines. Improper elimination is the cause of many problems. Heart and circulation are affected. By improving circulation, one can eliminate arthritis and cramps. Postures affect the functions of the liver, kidneys, pancreas, spleen, and reproduction organs of males and females. Control of breath and lungs is used with each and every position.

Back and Spine Most postures affect the spine and remove obstructions from that area. This helps free the nerve current flowing from the spine. By toning the spinal column, one improves the functioning of the entire body. Back problems are reduced. One's youthfulness is determined by the flexibility of the spine, and this flexibility is maintained through Yoga postures. Correction of spinal conditions will affect posture, walking, balance of the body, and proper breathing.

Weight and Muscle Tone Most positions provide the necessary stretch which is needed to tone the deep muscles. Yoga helps in establishing a healthy weight without going on a diet. The shoulderstand and other postures which affect the thyroid gland secretions, normalize weight problems. Overactive thyroid (excessive production of thyroxin hormones) makes one nervous and underweight, while an underactive thyroid produces an overweight problem. Yoga affects the metabolic functions of the body, burns up calories, and avoids overweight problems. When one feels relaxed and calm through postures and breathing, craving for food diminishes, and the body chooses only healthy food which helps in controlling weight problems. Also, craving for stimulants like smoking and alcohol diminish, which helps in controlling bad habits.

Emotional Balance Breathing and inverted positions like the headstand and shoulderstand control emotions and keep one calm and relaxed. Endocrine glands also control emotions. Practice builds resistance against frequent colds, allergies, and infections by keeping the entire body free from emotional shocks. Yoga practice brings emotional balance and freedom from mood swings and daily stress. This balance produces inner peace and creative energy.

Longevity Yoga practices purify the body, harmonize the emotions, and preserve vital energy. This preserved energy keeps one youthful and healthy, adding extra productive years to life.

Grass always looks greener at a distance. It is tempting to want to be in someone's shoes. Only when we let go of fantasies and accept ourselves do we see the truth with a clear vision and then progress will be made. Dharma means spontaneously being and acting in the present. Liberation comes from following our own Dharma no matter how low or insignificant it may seem.

Sometimes we know something, think about it, and believe that we are doing it. Food satisfies the stomach not by looking at it but by eating it. It becomes a mental habit to create an image of ourselves which is far from reality. The greater the distance between our self-image and expectations from reality the greater will be the conflict, guilt, and confusion.

Set your ultimate goal and maintain clarity of it. Believe in it, deserve and accept it and other faculties will follow in action to provide the results. Keep your eyes on the ultimate goal, the means may change. Take a detour when hindrance comes. Do not hang onto the means. Being attached to the means may result in forgetting the ultimate goal. Also, consider failures as a means to an end like a child learning to walk falls many times before he finally learns.

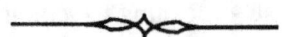

5

YOGA POSITIONS

GETTING READY

Sleeping, Waking, Cleansing Sleep is essential for rejuvenation. One should go to sleep around 9 to 10 P.M. and awake around 4 to 5 A.M. This allows maximum rest and rejuvenation. One should get six to eight hours of sleep depending upon age and activities. A hard mattress is healthy for the back. Sleeping position should be on the back or either side rather than the stomach, as sleeping on the stomach interferes with breathing and digestion. Fresh air should be circulating throughout the room. Say prayers, chant the Guru mantra, and surrender yourself to the Divine Lord before going to sleep. Dismiss worries or excitement from your mind, as they produce dreams and drain energy.

Rhythmic breathing is recommended for those who have problems falling asleep. Try to form regular sleeping and waking habits. Even if you can't go to sleep at a definite time, wake up at the same time. When this habit is developed, you will be able to wake up easily and feel rested. Wake up gently by stretching your body like an animal. Learn the techniques from your teacher. Don't rush and shock your nerves by jumping out of bed.

After waking up, brush your teeth, clean your tongue, rinse your eyes, and drink a large glass of lukewarm water. Clean your sinus passages with a saline solution. (These techniques are described in Chapter 23, Cleansing.) Now lie down on each side for two minutes which will ensure fast and proper elimination. Next, take a shower and put on fresh clothes.

There are six purification techniques (Shad kriyas) in Yoga:

1. Neti - Cleaning the nostril passage.
2. Dhauti - Cleaning the esophagus and stomach.
3. Basti - Cleaning the colon

4. Tratak - External concentration on a candle flame, described in Chapter 9, Concentration and Meditation.
5. Kapalbhati - Cleansing breathing, described in Chapter 6, Breathing.
6. Nauli - Churning the abdominal muscles, described later in this chapter.

Stretching and Limbering Practice the following stretches for limbering and relaxation. Learn properly from your teacher:
1. NECK ROLL: Relax the neck muscles with mental suggestion; let the head feel heavy until it starts hanging. Let it rotate clockwise and then counterclockwise. Dizziness and cracking noises are common in the beginning. This will stop after regular lubrication. This movement removes tension headaches and clears the head by promoting circulation in the brain.
2. ROCKING: Clasp your hands around the knees. Rock on your back with the rhythm of breathing. Keep your back rounded. This relaxes the back muscles and rejuvenates the spine.
3. EYES: Keep your eyes wide open and rotate them in a clockwise and counterclockwise direction. Rub your palms together and place them over your face. This exercise is good for the eyes, while the palming removes tension from the face and relaxes facial muscles. Use caution if you are wearing contact lenses.
4. ARMS and LEGS: Stretch out on your back, interlock your fingers and stretch your entire body in opposite directions as you inhale, trying to lengthen your body including the spine. Let go with exhalation. Next, in a sitting position, stretch your arms out to the sides, spread your fingers apart and then close your fists tightly. Do this several times. Rotate the fists and then the entire arm. Stretch the legs in front of you. Raise one leg at a time, stretch the foot forward, backwards, and then rotate the ankle joint in both directions without bending the knee. Practice squatting on your tip toes and then on flat feet. Fold your palms behind your back in the greeting gesture.
5. SWAN: Lie on the stomach with bent arms at the sides, rise up until arms are straight, and arch back giving the entire spine a good backwards stretch. Next, return to the knees and pull straight back into a kneeling position. Do this posture several times for good overall stretch. See Figures 1 and 2.

When stretching and limbering exercises are completed rest on your back with deep abdominal breathing.

BENEFITS: Stretching and limbering exercises prepare one for Hatha Yoga. They remove tension from deep muscles and rejuvenate them by improving circulation. They remove calcium deposits, and arthritis is reduced or prevented. These exercises also tone the nerves and the spine, and provide better sleep.

POSTURES
(For detailed pictures, variations, and benefits of all postures, see Hatha Yoga Practice Manual.)

Shoulderstand, Plough, Bridge, and Fish
Lie down on your back, relax with a few deep breaths, slowly raise the legs and back and come to the position in Figure 3. Hold this position as long as is comfortable and then slowly let the legs drop down in back of the head as shown in Figure 4, plough position. Again, hold for a comfortable time then return to shoulderstand. From shoulderstand go down on the back and then go into bridge position as in Figure 5. Then allow the body to stretch out on the floor and go into fish position, arching the upper back and neck as shown in Figure 6. Rest afterwards for an equal amount of time with recharging breathing. (See Chapter 6, Breathing.) Spend 3 to 6 minutes for entire shoulderstand routine.

Avoid the shoulderstand if you have a cold or infection in the eyes, ears, or throat. The shoulderstand routine is ideal for rejuvenating the body. This routine improves the nervous system and circulation, and also results in weight control. The plough posture tones up the sympathetic nervous system and gives orthopedic exercise to the spine, making it flexible and strong. Bridge posture strengthens and relaxes back muscles. Fish posture is complementary to shoulderstand and should be practiced at the end. It relaxes the neck area and helps correct bad posture.

Head-to-Knee
Sit with your legs stretched out in front of you. Arms rest on the legs. With inhalation raise your arms, drop the head back gently, and hold. With exhalation slowly lower the arms and upper body until the hands reach the toes. (Figure 7) Hold the breath out. While holding the toes, straighten up and

lengthen the spine (Figure 8). Feel the stretch throughout the body. Bend forward a second time to come to head-to-knee. With inhalation raise the arms once more and then exhale while lowering the arms slowly. Rest on your back with deep breathing. All forward bending positions affect the abdominal region. They improve digestion and elimination and provide an internal massage to vital internal organs. They limber the spine and make one flexible and youthful. You may modify the position by bending the knees.

Bow

Stretch out on the floor on the stomach with arms straight out in front of you. Bend the knees and grasp the feet or ankles with the hands, raising the head and arching the body. Now stretch the legs up and out, pulling the arms and upper body gently. As you become limber with this posture you may rock forward and backward. Inhale as you raise the body, and exhale as you gently lower the body. When you are finished, rest on your back with deep breathing. Backward bending positions are beneficial for strengthening the back and spinal column, and for removing backaches. They expand the lung capacity and improve breathing. (See Figures 9 and 10.) Modify by grasping one foot at a time with the opposite or the same hand.

Twist

Take a deep breath while straightening the body. With exhalation twist on one side, around your waist. Return with inhalation and repeat on the other side. Twist affects the spinal column, back muscles, and shoulders. It shapes the waist and massages the deep abdominal muscles and inner vital organs. (See Figure 11.)

Lion and Abdominal Lift

Lion posture is good for cleansing. Stand or kneel with legs apart. Rest your hands on the bent knees. Inhale deeply and exhale forcefully. At the same time, extend the tongue out as far as possible. Open the mouth and eyes wide and spread the fingers apart until the entire body stiffens. To derive the full benefits of lion posture, one should coordinate all of these movements simultaneously and visualize all of the impurities being thrown out. This posture should be done with an empty stomach. Lion is beneficial for cleansing the lungs, exercising the deep abdominal muscles, and improving circulation in the throat (which removes sore throat in the initial stages). It is also good for facial beauty and facial muscles. (See Figure 12.)

For the abdominal lift, take a cleansing breath and exhale forcefully holding the breath out. While holding the breath out, relax abdominal muscles and let them form a hollow cavity in the stomach. After mastering this you can practice moving stomach muscles in and out or churning them (nauli). Do these postures with an empty stomach and learn properly from a teacher. They are good cleansing positions and affect deep abdominal muscles. Digestion and elimination are improved, and abdominal muscles are strengthened. These postures also help in awakening Kundalini. (See Figure 13.)

Mudras

After purifying the body and mind through asanas (postures) and pranayamas (breathing techniques-Chapter 6), one practices mudras for awakening the spiritual force called Kundalini.

Mudra means to seal, to close, or to lock. Various techniques of mudras involve locking the prana within the body to awaken Kundalini.

Many postures like headstand and shoulderstand are also mudras. In practicing postures, one uses the body with mental effort, but in mudras prana moves the body while the mind remains a passive witness. Mudra also means gestures. Mudras become expressions of prana through body movements. Advanced students should practice Yoga positions with awareness of prana so that postures become meditative mudras. Mudras are retained for a very long time, while restricting prana and directing it for Kundalini awakening.

Lotus - Meditation - Relaxation

Place the left foot on the right thigh and the right foot on the left thigh. Keep the spine erect and the position evenly balanced. Rest your arms in your lap or your knees. This position is used for meditation. (See Figure 14.) Modify by using any comfortable sitting position. Practice cleansing breathing as described in Chapter 6, Breathing. Meditate on the flow of breath, remaining passive. Rest on the back and follow the relaxation technique as described in Chapter 7, Relaxation.

All of these positions may be modified to suit individual needs. The important thing to remember is to do them gently, slowly, with eyes closed, and with a meditative state of mind. Hold each position as long as is comfortable to get maximum stretch, doing proper breathing throughout.

Learn forbearance from <u>Earth</u>. Let your presence be soothing and purifying like <u>Water</u>. Like <u>Fire</u> which purifies pure metals from ore, let your austerities purify your consciousness from contamination. Like <u>Air</u> which is not attached to good or bad odors, remain unattached to the dualities of life. Like <u>Ether</u> that pervades the whole universe, remain aware of the divine essence permeating all living creatures.

Be like an ocean which remains calm as rivers throw more water or no water into it. The ocean does not overflow or dry up. Absorb the dualities of life without losing your inner peace.

Let your virtues spread by your own presence instead of pretence or speech. The fragrance of a flower spreads on its own. A candle lights up one room at a time while the sun lights up the universe.

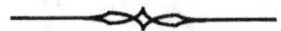

It is easy to join new groups, also to rebel against new ideas and to become joiners and quitters. No effort is required. It takes a brave person to accept challenge and experiment instead of simply accepting/rejecting.

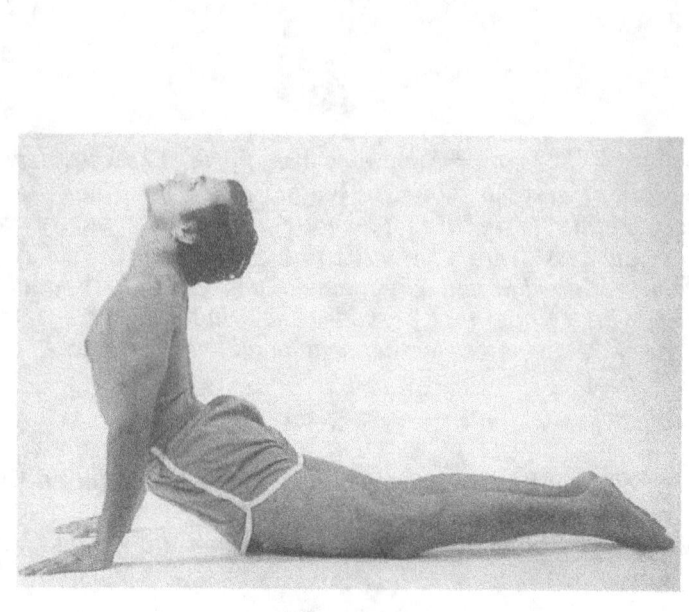

Figure 1

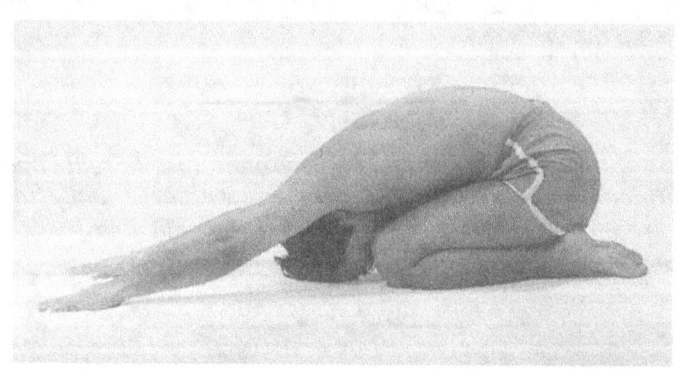

Figure 2
SWAN

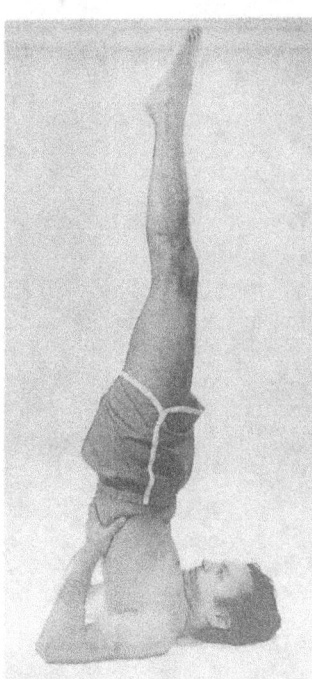

Figure 3 - SHOULDERSTAND

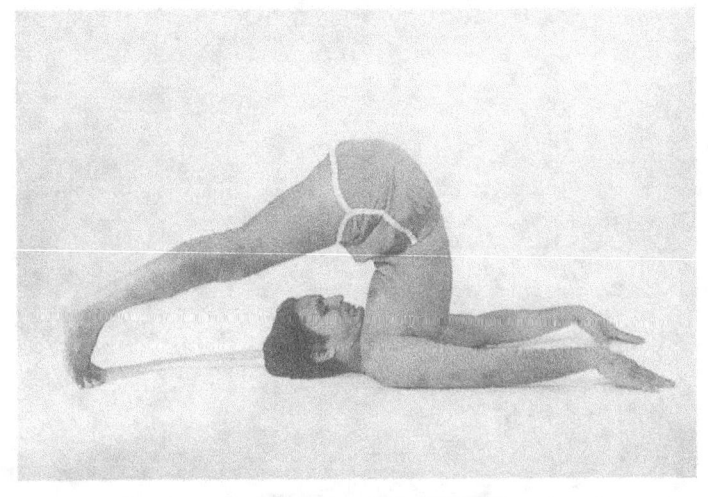

Figure 4 - PLOUGH

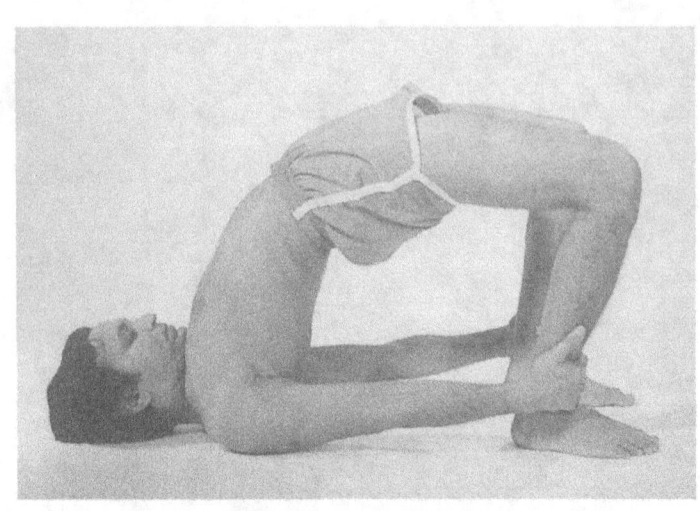

Figure 5 - BRIDGE

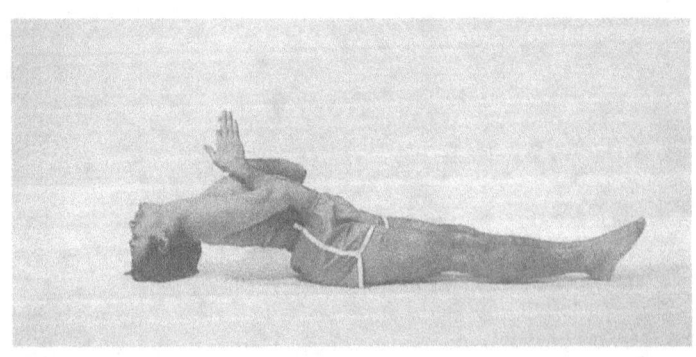

Figure 6 - FISH

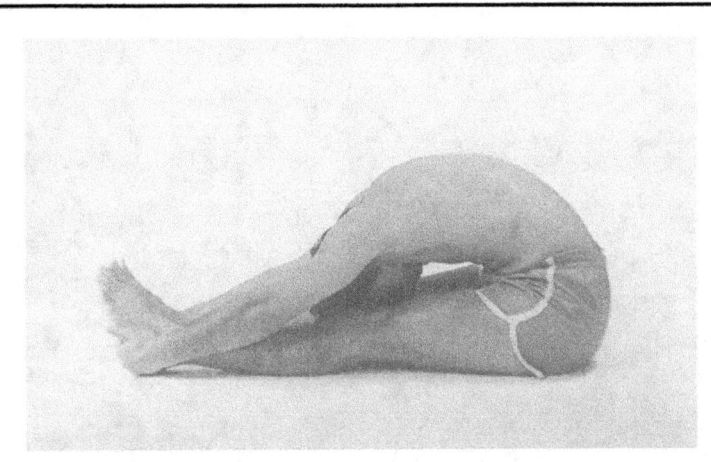

Figure 7

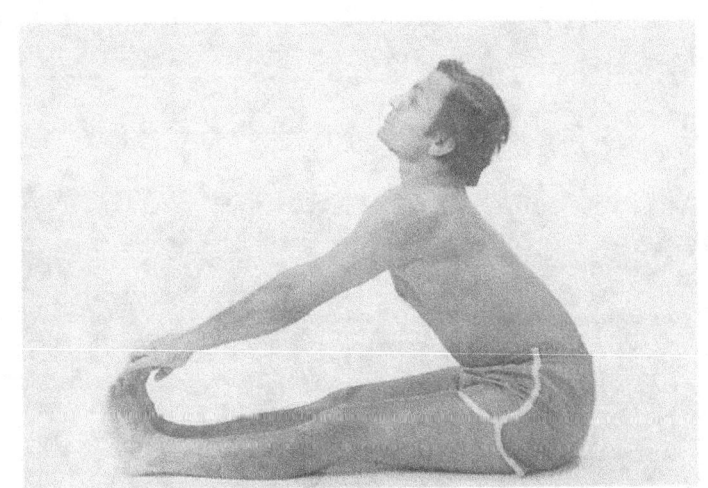

Figure 8

HEAD-to-KNEE

Yoga Positions

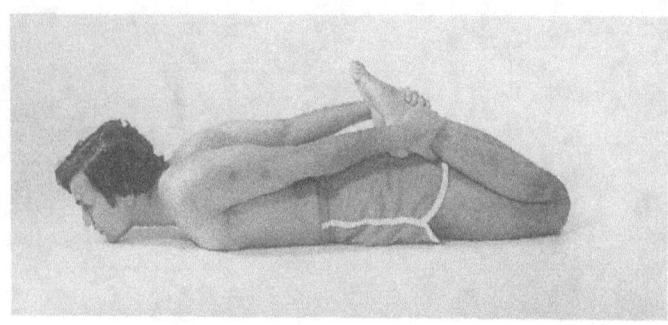

Figure 9

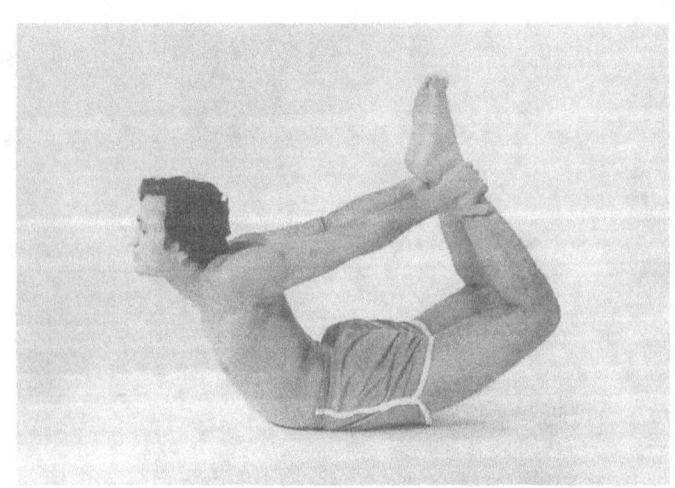

Figure 10

BOW

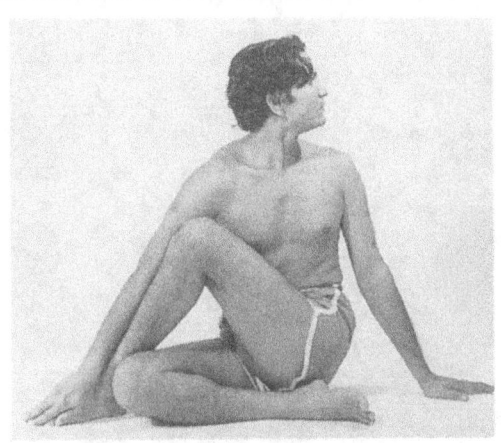

Figure 11 - TWIST

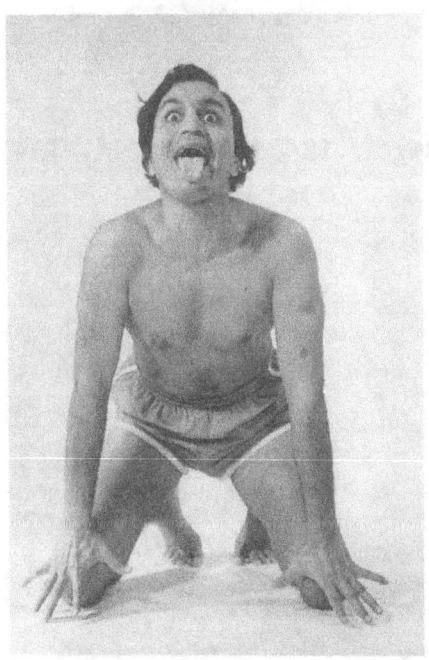

Figure 12 - LION

Yoga Positions

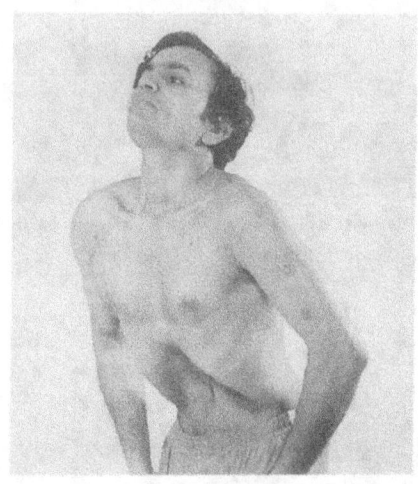

Figure 13 - ABDOMINAL LIFT

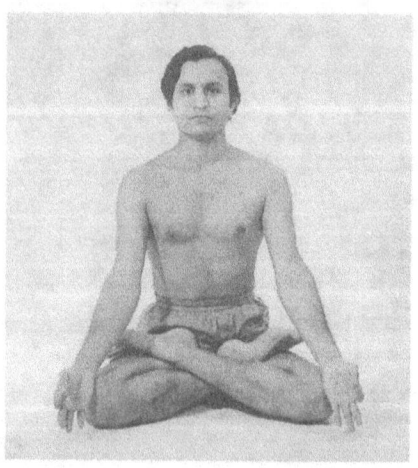

Figure 14 - LOTUS

6

BREATHING (PRANAYAMA)

Prana means vital life force or air, and Ayam means control. In the physical form pranayama is the technique of breath control. In the higher and subtler sense pranayama means control of the energy within our body and mind.

Physical sciences classify air as oxygen, carbon dioxide, nitrogen, etc., while Yoga defines prana (air) according to its functions within our body. There are five major and five minor pranas. The major pranas are Prana, Apana, Samana, Udana, and Vyana. They control the major vital functions of the body. The minor pranas control secondary functions of the body.

FUNCTIONS OF BREATH Breath is life. Breathing is the most vital function of our existence. Physically speaking, breathing provides oxygen and nourishment to the blood and removes carbon dioxide. It also regulates the pH of the blood and the water content of the body. We can survive without food for months and can survive without water for days, but we cannot survive without breathing even for a few minutes.

All living beings breathe constantly whether they are awake or asleep, conscious or unconscious. Why should one learn to breathe properly? The answer is obvious. Our physical and mental vitality are proportional to our breathing capacity and the rhythm of our breathing. Emotional states are related to our breathing. A peaceful condition of the mind produces rhythmic breathing, while an excited and disturbed condition of the mind produces erratic breathing. Inversely, our emotional states can be controlled by breathing. Our life span is determined by the number of breaths, not by the number of years. By mastering breathing, we can increase our life span and improve the quality of our life.

BREATHING MECHANISM As we inhale, air enters through the nasal passages, then passes through the pharynx, larynx, trachea, bronchus, bronchial tubes, and finally reaches alveoli (air sacks). It resembles an upside down tree. The nose is the roots, the bronchus is the trunk, the bronchial tubes are branches, and alveolis are the leaves. Air must reach all the way to the air sacks and fill them to provide proper nourishment, like a tree providing nourishment to the leaves.

Lungs are spongy and porous and their tissues are elastic. They are connected at the top by bronchis and are loose on the sides. The bottom of the lungs hang on the diaphragm.

The lungs are covered by numerous tiny blood capillaries which carry the blood to the heart. Impure blood is carried from the heart to the lungs via the veins, and the purified blood is carried by the arteries from the lungs to the heart.

Oxygen combines with hemoglobin in the blood and is circulated through the entire body, nourishing and replacing cells. The diaphragm controls the motion of the lungs. It is the muscular partition with a dome shape turned upward and separates the abdominal and thoracic cavities. It is an involuntary organ which can be made semi-voluntary by practice and will. It constantly moves up and down and controls our breathing. When the diaphragm moves down, it creates a vacuum in the lungs and allows air to rush into the lungs. When it moves up, it contracts the lungs pushing the air out.

When we inhale we saturate the alveoli. Each tiny alveoli is surrounded by tiny blood capillaries. The pressure difference allows oxygen to diffuse from the air sacks (alveoli) to the blood capillaries. Deep breathing provides more oxygen transfer to the blood.

Understanding the above description of the breathing mechanism enables students to learn to control their breathing. Control of the breath comes from the diaphragm and not from the lungs.

WRONG BREATHING Avoid the following ways of wrong breathing: 1. Do not try to move the shoulders and back to intake more air. The shoulder and chest muscles have no part in proper breathing. 2. Avoid chest and high breathing where an effort is made to fill the top part of the lungs. 3. Keep the mouth closed all the time, using the nostrils. Nasal passages have cilia and mucus to filter the air and provide a longer passage which allows the air to warm up and increase its moisture content before entering the lungs. Using the mouth for breathing exposes you to germs which may cause cold and infections. 4. An empty stomach is helpful for breathing. Girdles, belts, and tight clothing hinder breathing.

BEGINNER'S BREATHING (Abdominal or diaphragmatic breathing) Beginners should follow these suggestions to master their breathing in stages. It may take several weeks to master all the stages and develop good rhythm and coordination in your breathing.

1. Lie down comfortably on your back, place one hand on the abdominal region, close your eyes and relax. With no effort, notice and witness the movement of your abdominal muscles. You will notice that the abdominal muscles rise on inhalation and drop with exhalation. With inhalation the diaphragm drops down pushing the abdominal muscles out; with exhalation the diaphragm moves up creating a suction which tends to pull in the abdominal muscles.

One should master this first step before going any further. This is the rhythm of nature. We want to coordinate our forces with this rhythm. Many people do exactly the opposite type of breathing due to habit and as taught so prevalently in America. It will take extra effort to break this habit. Try to avoid excessive force which will tend to disturb the rhythm. Calmly witness and fall in tune with the movement in order to progress.

This breathing is called abdominal or diaphragmatic breathing. When you get used to the rhythm, let the abdominal muscles rise higher and drop lower to make your breathing become deeper and longer while maintaining the rhythm with the diaphragm.

2. Now try the second stage where your mouth is closed and your nostrils are used in breathing. The nostrils do not expand or contract but remain inactive and act as a passage. Concentrate on the back of your throat in the pharyngeal region and let a sound come from this area. This sound may be a smooth hissing which may or may not be audible. As long as your nostrils are inactive and you feel the cold air passing through the throat you are doing it right.

If you have any problem mastering the sound, pretend you are snoring but make it more silent and smooth. Using the pharynx like this is very valuable in producing relaxation and also helps to control the rhythm and length of your breathing. This sound of breathing is made while practicing the various postures. When you master step No. 2, coordinate it with step No. 1.

3. Counting: Begin timing your inhalation and exhalation with a uniform mental count. Establish a 1:1 ratio for inhalation to exhalation. Use the pharynx for controlling the duration of your breathing. You can contract your pharynx and control the length of your breath after a few weeks of practice. When you have mastered this rhythm, practice retention of the breath by contracting the throat muscles. Hold it comfortably. Establish a 2:1:2 ratio for inhalation, retention, and exhalation. Do not hold the breath beyond your capacity. If you have to rush and force your exhalation, you are doing it beyond your capacity. There should be no retention of breath after exhalation.

Combine the three steps above and practice from ten to thirty rounds (inhalation, retention, and exhalation together make one round) with an empty stomach in the morning and in the evening, or at least once during the day. In the beginning it may make you slightly dizzy due to the sudden supply of oxygen to the brain. Increase the number of counts in your breathing while maintaining the same ratio. An increase in the number of counts will indicate progress in your breathing capacity. During the day remain aware of your breathing. While walking, coordinate your breath with your steps.

YOGIC BREATHING This breathing involves filling the lungs from bottom to top by using diaphragmatic/abdominal breathing, then mid-breathing, and finally high breathing in a continuous flowing manner. This fills the entire area of the lungs. Practicing Yogic Breathing regularly will activate the unused portions of your lungs, and your breathing will be deeper and more rhythmic during the day and during sleep even though you are not conscious of it. After practicing this Yogic or Beginner's Breathing, you will find it easier to coordinate breathing with Yoga positions.

Technique: Sit in a lotus or cross legged position with the back straight and the spine vertical. You will have direct control of the diaphragm now and won't need to manipulate the abdominal muscles. Make your breathing smooth and steady, without pulses or hesitations.

Keep your back and shoulders relaxed and motionless. Fill up the lungs from bottom to top. Mental visualization will help the control of breathing. After the lungs are filled to the top visualize them expanding to the sides. At this stage let the chest expand forward without moving the body, and exhale in the exact reverse order.

WALKING BREATHING Practice walking breathing when you take a regular daily walk. Walking is an excellent exercise that anyone can do. You may walk at a slow or a faster speed, or use a combination of both, but keep it uniform for the rhythmic counts required in Walking Breathing. Count mentally with each step 1, 2, 3, 4, etc. at your own rate while breathing in, and then count 1, 2, 3, 4 as you breathe out. Keep a 1:1 ratio of breathing in to breathing out. You may retain the breath after breathing in using a 2:1:2 ratio. 1, 2, 3, 4 breathe in - 1, 2, retain - 1, 2, 3, 4 breathe out. Keep the body aligned and use correct posture to derive maximum benefits. Utilize and be aware of breathing while walking, climbing steps, lifting any object, swimming, jogging, or other activities. It will rejuvenate you instead of making you tired.

RHYTHMIC BREATHING Rhythmic breathing can be practiced after one has mastered beginner's breathing. Beginner's breathing should be mechanical and automatic so that one's mind is free to do rhythmic breathing.

Stretch out on your back. Place one hand on your stomach. Become aware of your abdominal, diaphragm, and lung movements. Feel the rhythm. Place the other hand over the heart and observe the rhythm of your heart.

Allow your breathing and heart beats to synchronize. Count your heart beats mentally as you breathe in, allow one count for pause, count while breathing out, then one count for pause. Keep the rhythm that suits you. (It will be close to a 1:1 ratio.) Let the process absorb your total attention. After mastering the technique, you may feel the internal rhythm and can practice this breathing anywhere and anytime, using mental counts if desired. You may not need to place your hands on the stomach or chest.

Remember, rhythm is more important than the length of your breath. Use a fewer number of counts than your capacity in order to maintain the rhythm for a long time without getting tired. Determine the number of counts you want to use with each breath and tune up your mind in counting and watching your breath. This breathing will take you to a state of deep relaxation.

The heart and lungs are the flywheels which start all the motions in our body. By coordinating them, all other organs become coordinated and fall in rhythm, which produces deep relaxation and thus provides optimum conditions for healing to take place in the body and mind. One establishes rhythm in the body, then rhythm of body and mind, and finally the rhythm of individual self with the whole universe. When one feels harmony and peace, loneliness disappears.

Rhythmic breathing is ideal for controlling and eventually eliminating insomnia, restlessness of the mind, and improving concentration. It is perfectly normal if you fall asleep while doing rhythmic breathing.

RECHARGING BREATHING Recharging breathing can be practiced after mastering beginner's breathing. Rest on your back or sit in lotus position with palms touching the feet to complete the circuit of energy. Do deep breathing with retention until it becomes effortless and mechanical. While the physical breathing is carried on by the sub-conscious mind, let your mind visualize and experience the following recharging process:

As you inhale, visualize the vital energy (prana) entering your lungs; with each retention visualize prana penetrating the deep muscles and nerves, recharging and healing them. As you exhale, visualize all the tensions, anxieties, physical and mental impurities being expelled in the form of dark smoke. With retention you can direct prana to any area in need of healing. Visualize the body to be porous like a sponge. As you breathe in, feel the expansion and swelling. As you breathe out, experience the squeeze or contraction.

Feel the pores enlarging as you breathe through them until the inside and outside atmosphere become homogeneous. Dissolve your physical boundaries; let the mind dissolve into universal mind. Experience your existence as Being. Merge and identify with each thought, each object, and each sensation as happens naturally. This breathing is ideal for recharging, healing, and vitalizing both body and mind.

HEALING BREATHINGS

Self-Rejuvenation: Sit cross-legged in a comfortable position. Let both hands cover both feet. Practice basic rhythmic breathing passively, counting mentally a 1:1 ratio until the mind dissolves.

Prana radiates through the palms and the feet during the process. Touching palms and feet completes the energy cycle which will rejuvenate you as energy accumulates. Be aware of the energy flow cycling through your body. It will provide a lift during low feelings in energy or enthusiasm.

Solar Plexus: The solar plexus is called the abdominal brain. It is located in the back in the pit of the stomach below the navel on each side of the spine. A mass of sympathetic nerves and ganglia are located here. It is a storehouse of prana and one can draw energy by focusing on this center. The martial arts use this center for inner balance and strength.

Self-Healing-General: Breathe in prana. Retain the breath and focus on the solar plexus. As you breathe out feel the prana shooting out through the nerve channels reaching each and every part of your body. Visualize the tiny sparks of prana at the nerve endings. Feel the subtle vibrations of prana shaking off the impurities, and feel the entire body vibrating. At the end, mentally retain the desired image of your health and peace. This image will become reality in time.

Self-Healing-Specific: Rest in a comfortable position. Practice rhythmic breathing. When you get in rhythm, visualize that you are breathing in prana from the universal source. Take the prana to the solar plexus. Retain, and feel the prana building up in this area.

As you breathe out, feel the prana rising from the solar plexus to the right arm and flowing down to the palm and fingertips. Then place your hand on the area you want to heal. Feel the warmth transmitted from your fingers to this area. Keep up with several breaths. Then place the hand on the next area.

For the relief of pain in a specific area, apply the above technique the first time where prana is taken to the solar plexus, then to the area of pain. The second time take in prana with an incoming breath, no retention, and breathe out directly to the area of pain as if you are blowing the pain away. Repeat several times. Remain passive and experience the harmony of prana flowing throughout the entire body.

To heal others use the same techniques. Be a channel and feel the energy flowing through you. At the end of the session, shake and wash your hands.

Group Healing: Each person in the group should practice rhythmic breathing individually until everyone finds his inner rhythm. Extend both arms and hold hands, making a completely closed circle of energy. Chant OM continuously for several minutes.

Feel the collective energy circulating through the circle in a wave, flowing through your body, healing it. Also, feel the expansion of your consciousness as your OM chant merges into the total OM vibrations.

Distant Healing: At this time you can send healing group energy to any person or persons you desire to heal. Think of this person, visualize his image. Look at a picture or form the image by description. Feel his nearness and send your love by becoming an open channel. Prana knows no boundary or distance. It travels and provides energy to the person in need of healing. It helps if the person being healed can synchronize the time, and remain open and receptive at that moment.

CLEANSING BREATHINGS

Kapalbhati: Kapal means skull and bhati means shines. Kapalbhati purifies the brain and shines the skull. It is one of the cleansing practices (kriyas) of Hatha Yoga.

Sit properly with the spine vertical. Quickly and forcefully exhale through the nostrils without moving the body. Pull the abdominal muscles in allowing the diaphragm to lift up, which contracts the lungs for thorough exhalation. Relax at the end, and the diaphragm will fall back allowing inhalation to take place automatically.

There is no retention of breath in this breathing. This process of inhalation and exhalation is carried on rapidly using one's own rhythm. Exhalation is forceful while inhalation is passive. Do fifteen to thirty expulsions at a time, or until you feel a slight dizziness. This is one round. Do two to three rounds with a pause between each round. Increase the number of expulsions per round according to your capacity. One can practice a hundred or more expulsions per round in the advanced stages.

Beginners may use the mouth for exhalation instead of the nostrils, but inhalation is always done through the nostrils. It is important not to move the body while doing this breathing; instead, establish better control of the diaphragm. Also, maintain your individual rhythm of breathing.

CAUTION: This breathing oxygenates the brain suddenly and may cause dizziness. With regular practice, the brain is able to absorb more oxygen and this problem is overcome. Stop this breathing as soon as you feel dizzy; close your eyes and experience the after-effect.

If possible, practice this breathing outdoors, or open the windows so that fresh air penetrates the lungs.

Bhastrika: Bhastrika means bellows. The lungs do the pumping movement like the bellows of a blacksmith. One should attempt Bhastrika after mastering Kapalbhati. This technique involves forceful exhalation and forceful inhalation through the nostrils. It is more vigorous, and the entire respiratory system is involved in the breathing instead of the diaphragm only. At the end of several expulsions take a deep breath and hold it according to your capacity. In the advanced stages, or after longer practices, one may apply three locks. These are explained under Anuloma-Viloma Pranayama.

Benefits of Cleansing Breathing
Kapalbhati is a cleansing practice, while Bhastrika is a pranayama. They are practiced for different purposes, yet they have similarities in technique and benefits. Following are some of the common benefits of these breathing practices:

Under normal breathing conditions, our diaphragm moves slightly, allowing some impure air to be pushed out and replacing it with fresh air. This leaves a large portion of residual air within the lungs. The only way this residual air can be removed is by force.

Successive expulsions remove most of the congested impure air and replace it with fresh air (oxygen). This allows oxygen to penetrate the air sacks, activating unused air sacks and unused portions of the lungs. More oxygen is provided to the blood stream, which nourishes the entire body and brain.

One can feel the opening of the congested nostrils and throat and feel the cool air penetrating throughout the lungs. Spasms are removed from the bronchial tubes and asthma conditions are helped. One feels a tingling sensation throughout the body due to cellular oxygenation. The body feels weightless, and a floating sensation results.

In addition, the brain receives a richer supply of blood and the mind feels quiet. It increases concentration by removing restless thoughts from the mind. Ideally, these breathing techniques are practiced before meditation. They provide more oxygen to the blood stream and delay the generation of carbon dioxide pressure. This suspends one's breathing which produces a transcendental state.

These breathing techniques remove impurities from the lungs and increase lung capacity. By satisfying the lungs and respiratory organs with oxygen, cravings for wrong food and smoking are reduced. A few rounds of these techniques will clear your head from confusion, and you will be instantly rejuvenated. It will give you the feeling of taking an internal bath. At the end of mental activities these breathing techniques would be very refreshing.

Cleansing breathing techniques are different from hyperventilation. Hyperventilation is an involuntary pattern of breathing disturbance, while cleansing breathing is voluntary and is a controlled breathing to oxygenate the entire body quickly and thoroughly for positive benefits.

Bhastrika pranayama is very effective for awakening Kundalini (psychic powers located within the spinal column).

ANULOMA VILOMA PRANAYAMA
(Alternate nostril breathing)

Anuloma Viloma Pranayama is a major pranayama for advanced students. There are many other pranayamas for specific benefits. Anuloma Viloma Pranayama will bring the most benefit if practiced daily. This is such a major pranayama that traditionally the word pranayama refers to Anuloma Viloma Pranayama. With regular practice of this technique, as guided by a teacher, it will open the gates of higher practices of Yoga.

Pranayama stabilizes prana, without which concentration and meditation is impossible. Traditional practices of concentration and meditation widely practiced by the masses are of a low category because prana has not been mastered. Mastery of this pranayama may take several months to several years of intensive full time practice.

Our spine is called Meru Dunda (supporting pole) which sustains our life. We have an astral body which is the exact counterpart of our gross body. It contains the spine and the network of the nervous system. These astral nerves are called the nadis. There are three major and 72,000 minor nadis. The Shushumna is the central nadi located within the astral spine.

The Shushumna connects the seven chakras (psychic centers within the spine). The average person's Shushumna is clogged.

Yoga practices open up the nadis and allow prana to flow through them. Prana pierces the chakras, opens up one's consciousness, and cultivates psychic powers. The average person may, from time to time, get a spark of higher consciousness when some prana travels through the Shushumna (as a result of meditation, drugs, or other means). This is called Pranotthana (raising of prana). Kundalini is considered awakened only when the chakras are pierced. It takes years of diligent practice to awaken Kundalini.

On the left side of the Shushumna there is a major nadi called Ida, which has lunar or cooling qualities. Breathing through the left nostril utilizes the Ida nadi. The major nadi on the right side of the spine is called Pingala, which has solar or stimulating qualities. Breathing through the right nostril utilizes the Pingala nadi.

If a person breathes only through the left nostril by blocking his right nostril, it will cool down his physiological activities by reducing blood pressure, slowing down nervous activity, and lowering body temperature. When one uses only the right nostril, while blocking the left, he can stimulate and accelerate all the above physiological functions.

In a healthy person only one nostril is active at a time, while the other is partially blocked. The other nostril becomes activated after approximately two hours. This process of alternating the nostrils every two hours regulates the anabolic and catabolic activities in the body. In a sick person the rhythm of this breathing becomes upset.

The duration of each nostril's activeness also depends upon the time of day, the season, and other factors. Alternate nostril breathing cleans and purifies the Ida and Pingala nadis, so that the middle nadi, Shushumna, becomes activated. In samadhi, only the Shushumna is active while the other two nadis are inactive. Dawn and dusk are the rhythmic times when there is rhythm in the body and both nostrils function at the same time allowing the Shushumna to be activated. This is why yogis recommend meditation at these times.

Technique: Sit in a lotus or cross leg position, keeping the spine, neck, and head in a vertical position. Close the right nostril with the thumb of your right hand. Place the last two fingers on the left nostril. Bend the middle two fingers or rest them on your forehead. Now loosen the fingers from your left nostril and inhale slowly through the left nostril. Immediately close the left nostril and exhale through the right one by lifting the thumb. Now, reverse the process by inhaling through the right nostril and exhaling through the left. In the beginning keep the ratio of your inhalation to exhalation 1:1 with no retention. Inhalation is called Poorak, and exhalation is called Rechaka, while retention is called Kumbhaka.

NOTE: In this breathing you have to use your nostrils directly. Do not use the pharynx for making the sound as is done in beginner's breathing. Inhalation should be gentle and smooth. Exhalation should be extremely gentle so there is no sound.

After mastering the 1:1 ratio, increase it to 1:2 ratio. Then gradually try retention of breath (Kumbhaka). Hold the breath in after inhalation. Do not hold after exhalation.

Gradually develop mastery of pranayama until at the highest stage of practice the ratio becomes 1:4:2 for inhalation, retention, and exhalation respectively. These three stages together make one round of pranayama. Practice ten to fifty rounds in each sitting. One may practice one, two, or three times during the day.

It may take about a year's practice for an average person to master the above stage. One may practice the following three bandhas (locks) as taught by an experienced teacher. In most cases the locks will happen automatically when one has purified his nadis.

Jalandhara Bandha (Chin Lock) While doing Kumbhaka (retention), press the chin firmly against the chest. This pulls the upper region of the spinal cord and pushes prana (located between the throat and heart chakra) downward.

Moola Bandha (Anus Lock) Press the perineum with a heel (Siddhasana, a meditative position) and contract the anus muscles. This helps to draw Apana (located between the anus and pelvis chakra) upward. It also helps in drawing the sexual energy for sublimation.

Uddiyana Bandha (Abdominal Lock) This is a Yoga position. Exhale thoroughly, hold the breath out, and contract the abdominal muscles inward. This affects the solar plexus.

Practicing these three bandhas unites prana and apana and opens the passage of Shushumna, which is a technique for awakening Kundalini. If a person forces himself in kumbhaka and the bandhas without purifying the nadis, impurities from the nadis will come out in the form of serious physical and mental diseases.

PREPARATION FOR PRANAYAMA

Observe the basic disciplines of Hatha Yoga. Along with these disciplines, make sure that purity of diet is maintained. Eat satvik (pure) food, eat less than hunger, and fast occasionally.

If you intend to take the practice of pranayama seriously you must observe celibacy, as explained under Yamas in Chapter 3, Raja Yoga. Celibacy provides the energy, while pranayama provides the heat. Like water which turns to steam upon heating, our sexual energy sublimates into creative energy with pranayama. Just as a container burns with excess heat when there is no water in it, the body gets into serious trouble when one practices pranayama without celibacy. Regular pranayama, however, without excessive retention and locks is safe for the average person.

BENEFITS

There are numerous general and specific benefits of basic breathing and advanced pranayamas. They can be summed up as follows:

Physical: Breathing provides oxygen to the red blood cells, and these cells nourish all the cells and tissues of the body. Our entire body is made of cellular structures. Proper breathing keeps the body firm by nourishing the muscles, preventing wrinkles. Muscles can then work for a longer time without becoming tired. By longer and deeper rhythmic breathing one extends his life span. Metabolic activities are controlled. Organs of digestion and elimination are also affected, increasing their efficiency. Breathing produces rhythm in the body and mind, which improves muscular and mental coordination, saving time and energy.

Mental: Our brain requires three times more oxygen than our body. Oxygen nourishes our brain and increases concentration and mental clarity. One can do more mental work without getting tired, and one needs less sleep.

Nervous System: The nervous system is closely connected with breathing. By slowing down the breath we can slow down emotional disturbances. Proper breathing brings instant control of our moods. We can eliminate anger and anxiety just by doing deep breathing. Insomnia, stress, tension, and headache problems can be controlled with breathing techniques. By controlling our negative emotions, energy is preserved.

Spiritual: In a higher sense, breathing controls our life force which can be utilized for healing ourselves or others. Pranayama helps in awakening Kundalini and in speeding up our spiritual evolution. Anuloma Viloma Pranayama controls anabolic and catabolic processes and establishes physical and mental harmony.

Habits: Breathing produces relaxation and satisfies the breathing passages, which helps in overcoming smoking habits. Breathing is successfully used in natural childbirth. It is soothing for the nerves and stops the craving for alcohol, candy, wrong foods, and overeating. Breathing increases resistance to disease and infection. Proper breathing also strengthens mental and physical endurance and will power.

Biofeedback: Breathing is a link between body and mind. Mastering breathing brings body and mind in closer communication with each other. One can control blood pressure, tension headaches, pain, and heal himself at will.

Longevity: We are how we breathe. The quality of our life and its longevity depend upon our breathing. Breathing opens us up to the greater potential within us. Creative energy unfolds using proper breathing techniques.

To master meditation you should change your life style, learn non-attachment, and simplify your life. A car that goes at 100 mph takes X minutes and Y feet before it can be stopped. Another car that travels at a slower speed can be stopped in a shorter amount of time and distance. A simpler and non-attached life style make it easier to meditate and to reach deeper levels more quickly.

7

RELAXATION

All machines need to be cooled off when they overheat. Our body is a very sensitive machine and needs proper rest. Without proper rest it loses its efficiency and can develop many problems. Nature has devised a system of rest by providing sleep to relax the body and the mind. Yet sleep may not provide proper relaxation if one's muscles are tense during sleep or one's mind revolves through restless dreams. One needs to learn the art of relaxation and sleep to rejuvenate his body. An average healthy person may need 6 to 8 hours of sleep. The best time to sleep is around 9 to 10 PM and to wake up around 4 to 5 AM. During this time one takes advantage of the rhythm of nature for a deep restful sleep. Many people lie in bed for hours and don't find any rest, or they may take a long vacation without success in relaxation. Long inactive hours will produce more tiredness in some people, while others work hard and are still more relaxed. If one masters the art of relaxation, he does not require a vacation because each day's activity becomes recreation and life itself becomes a vacation.

Relaxation and laziness look alike on the surface, yet in reality, they are quite different. Laziness is lack of energy and enthusiasm, while relaxation is controlled, channelized energy which is available for use at any time, and is under the individual's command. Relaxation converts restless energy into creative positive energy.

Most people are concerned about gaining more energy by eating healthy food and by other sources, while neglecting to check their outgoing energy. For example, if a person increases his expenses while earning a higher salary, he will still have no savings. Relaxation is the technique of checking and controlling outgoing energy. Tension is produced out of habits. Habits are automatic actions performed by our subconscious mind. The habit of relaxation can be formed by consciously working at it until it becomes subconscious and automatic. Constant awareness is the best technique of relaxation. One should keep check of his physical posture, mental and emotional states from time to time. Observance of children and pets can teach us a very good lesson in relaxation.

STAGES OF RELAXATION

There are several stages of relaxation. The process is inside out. The process of tension is generated from our ego (ahamkara or I consciousness) which reflects on our mental faculty, and mind directs energy (prana) to the physical body. The process of relaxation involves the reverse process of withdrawing from the body and mind and going towards the ego.

PHYSICAL RELAXATION

All physical activities produce muscular tension, drain energy, and can make one physically tired and exhausted. Persons without coordination and discipline make many unnecessary movements and become tired, while people who are skilled perform the same activity gracefully, without any exertion. People who are restless engage themselves in unnecessary parties, social activities, and drain their energy. Without the proper mental attitude and control, recreational activities also drain energy.

There are several techniques for producing physical relaxation.

1. **Awareness:** There is usually some tension in the muscles of the body. When one becomes aware, he can let tension release by itself. Catch yourself while sitting, walking, talking, and you will notice some tension in your back, hands, legs, face, etc. Notice also if there is any unnecessary movement of your arms or head. By being aware you can be free from these tensions. Tension can also be removed by watching the breath.

2. **Stretching:** Stretch and then let go. Yoga postures produce relaxation by using this technique. Stretching allows blood circulation in the deep muscles and by letting go they attain their normal relaxed position. Yogic massage involves specific massage to generate relaxation to various muscles of the body.

3. **Suggestion:** Make a mental suggestion and then withdraw energy. Any physical activity involves the subconscious or conscious mind directing prana to certain muscles. Relaxation is the reverse process where you withdraw the energy

from various muscles and organs; this produces instantaneous relaxation.

4. **Controlling Senses:** One can produce relaxation by controlling the energy which is going out through our senses. Five senses produce stimulus for our nerves and drain our energy. Watching TV and listening to the radio or tapes are means by which we drain our energy. Chapter 3, Raja Yoga, explains pratyahara which is control of the senses.

MENTAL RELAXATION

1. **Controlling Emotions:** Emotions drain our energy at a faster rate than the above means. Human have six detrimental emotions called Shad Ripu (six enemies). The six emotions are: desires (kama), anger (krodha), greed (lobha), pride (mada), passion (moha), and jealousy and hate (matsara). One should master these emotions to preserve energy. Anger for a moment will drain energy for hours and also upset digestion, nerves, breathing, and heart beat. In the same way, the other emotions drain our energy.

2. **Controlling Mind:** Mental activities drain more energy than physical activities. Worry and anxiety can produce constant drain at a subconscious level of mind. Persons may not perform any physical movements and may still become exhausted due to mental worry. Mental relaxation can be produced by the proper mental attitude towards life. (Read Chapter 17, Karma Yoga, for further details.) Work with interest and love, and then surrender the fruits of all actions to God. Generally speaking, proper breathing helps in producing mental relaxation and quiets the mind. Concentration produces mental relaxation by reducing scattered, distracting thoughts from the mind.

SPIRITUAL RELAXATION

Spiritual relaxation is relaxation of the highest kind. It involves transcendence and rising above the limitations and barriers of body and mind. In reality it is meditation. One removes the ego consciousness which keeps him separate from the rest of the universe. This separateness produces loneliness and fear. If there is no separateness, who will be afraid of whom? Deep-rooted tensions exist at this level, and without removing tension at the spiritual level, relaxation remains incomplete.

A TECHNIQUE OF RELAXATION

Before starting the relaxation technique, go through the following stretching exercises to allow the body to relax: neck roll, rocking, palming, and stretching of arms and legs.

Now lie down on your back in the shavasana (corpse) position for relaxation. The room should be comfortable and free from distractions. A thick carpet or mat is helpful. The mind should be free from rush and preoccupation. Unwind completely before starting the relaxation.

Interlock your fingers, invert your palms and stretch your arms and legs in opposite directions, trying to lengthen your entire body. Be sure to stretch and lengthen the spine also. Next, shake the arms, legs, and fingers, as if you were shaking water off them. Let the arms and legs fall aside comfortably. Roll the head from side to side, and let it rest on either side. Allow the facial muscles to relax by removing all expression and tension. Close the eyes without any strain, and let and eyelids relax. Be sure there is no tension in closing the mouth; let the lips relax and the jaws hang down with gravity. Let the mind be free from all thoughts of past and future. The past is a dream which is gone, while desires, expectations and worries about the future are imaginary. Tell the mind that it can think and worry as much as it wants after the relaxation.

Now start concentrating on various areas of the body. The torch light of awareness is strong enough to remove tension from deep muscles. It is not necessary to move any area of the body during this concentration. Mentally travel from the toes upward towards the feet, legs, thighs, buttocks, pelvic region, waist, stomach, back, chest, shoulders, upper arms, forearms, fingers, neck, throat, head, and face. Progress slowly at your own pace.

Concentrate on the surface muscles, then go deeper and let the awareness penetrate through deep muscles and nerves. As you go through the entire body, it will become relaxed and motionless. You will have no desire to move; still, you have complete freedom to move if you want to.

Feel very comfortable in this position. Let your senses be free from their respective objects. Even if you hear any noise, let it turn into soothing music to aid your relaxation. Don't fight distractions; recognize them and then ignore them. They will die away in the background by themselves.

Practice ten rounds of abdominal breathing. Then passively concentrate on your breath. Abdominal breathing allows you the freedom of breathing in rhythm. As you become aware of your breath, it will slow down and become shallow. As the breathing slows down, feel your heart slowing down its pumping action. As a result the heart and lungs, two basic flywheels of our life, will reduce metabolic processes, nerve activities, and will produce complete rhythm so there is a minimum of activity sustaining life. Breathing will become extremely slow to the point of suspension.

For the second time, travel through the body to insure further relaxation. Let the mind travel up with each inhalation, traveling from the toes to the top of the head, and with each exhalation, traveling down from the head to the toes. This time let the awareness reach the deeper areas, glands, joints, and involuntary muscles. Feel a cool current flowing with your awareness.

In a short time you will feel your body to be weightless and floating. Let this feeling grow. Feel that your body is not gross, but subtle vibrating molecules. Feel yourself to be like a weightless cloud, floating in the vast open sky, feeling freedom and peace. Or, you may transport your consciousness to the pleasant memory of some past experiences.

Now let yourself expand and merge with the environment and the objects around you. Merge with all the objects of the room, then expand beyond the boundaries of the room, eventually merging with the whole universe. Feel that you are existing everywhere in the universe and the whole universe is part of you.

This process will gradually dissolve your mind and lead you to a transcendental experience. Feel that you are without size and shape, time and space, free from weight, burdens, gains and loss, pleasures and pains, birth and death. Now affirm that you are pure consciousness, which is pure existence, pure consciousness, and pure bliss. Stay in this state as long as you like, experiencing bliss.

Come out of the relaxation very gently by gradually being aware of your breathing, heart beats, and environment, then stretch your toes, fingers, and the rest of your body.

BENEFITS OF RELAXATION

Relaxation has numerous benefits. It is the key to health and happiness. Physically, it removes tension and fatigue. It relaxes and produces clarity of mind. With a relaxed body and mind, one can perform more tasks with less tiredness. Tension, headaches, insomnia, etc. can be eliminated with the mastery of relaxation.

During relaxation the body temperature, blood pressure, and metabolic processes slow down, which provide rest for our internal organs and allow them to regenerate. Rhythm is produced in the entire body, which is the best condition for any kind of physical, mental, or emotional healing. During this time of harmony, blocks are removed from the path of prana. Prana penetrates through deep muscles and nerves, and provides healing.

Yogic relaxation produces alpha brain waves, a very creative state of mind. One can utilize this state for solving problems and developing new ideas.

Relaxation is one of the basic requirements for mastering meditation. Without the art of relaxation, one cannot progress in meditation.

In addition, relaxation increases one's awareness and openness. With these qualities one is able to see situations clearly, study his own life, and solve many problems with ease. The quiet state of mind produced by proper relaxation is very conducive to learning and absorbing more knowledge in a short amount of time.

When you encounter negative thoughts or face a person annoying you, arguing, or insulting you, etc., observe your breath for a few moments, observe silence, and do not argue. You will disassociate yourself for a few moments and miss the critical moment. Diffuse yourself like a wet match that does not ignite.

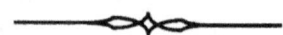

8

KUNDALINI YOGA

Our physical body has an identical counterpart in energy form which is called the Astral body. Our Astral body is controlled by astral nerves called nadis. This body contains ten major nadis from which 72,000 minor nadis spread throughout the astral body. Prana (the life force) flows through these nadis.

The Shushumna is the central nadi and corresponds to the spinal cord. Within this there are seven energy centers (chakras) which correspond to the nerve plexuses. The average person is a slave to Prakriti (nature) as their nadis are blocked. The goal of Yoga is to purify the minor nadis, then raise the energy through the Shushumna channel and awaken the energy centers (chakras) within it. As these chakras awaken, one attains spiritual consciousness. The final goal of Yoga is liberation where Prakriti (the lowest chakra) unites with Purusha (the highest chakra).

Yoga positions, yogic breathing, cleansing, fasting, and meditation are prerequisites for Kundalini. (See Chapter 9 for Kundalini Meditation techniques.) Kundalini awakens effortlessly with the above practices. One should not use any forceful techniques without guidance.

Kundalini Yoga is an ancient science. One should beware of frauds and myths concerning Kundalini Yoga. The chart on the following pages gives a description of the seven centers within the spine.

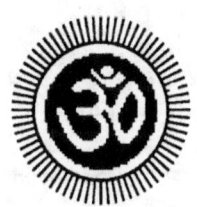

CHAKRA

CHAKRA	Location	Corresponding Plexus	Element	Organ of Perception
Sahasrara	Crown of Head	Pineal Gland	Shunyata (Void)	Transcends Senses
Agnya	Space Between Eyes	Cavernous Plexus	Mahat (Intuition)	Mental
Vishuddha	Base of Throat	Laryngeal Plexus	Ether	Sound and Hearing
Anahat	Heart	Cardiac Plexus	Air	Emotions (love) Touch
Manipura	Navel	Solar Plexus	Fire	Sight
Swadhishthana	Over Spleen	Prostatic Plexus	Water	Taste
Muladhara	Base of Spine	Sacral Plexus	Earth	Smell

No matter how much turmoil is in the world, our inner Self (Atman) always remains peaceful and tranquil. The eye of the hurricane is always calm.

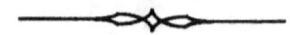

CHART

Bija	Devata	Color	Petals	Represents
--	Paramatma	Violet	Thousand Petals	Nirbij Samadhi
Aum	Atman	Indigo	Two Petals	Sabij Samadhi
Hum	Soul	Blue	Sixteen Petals	Awareness of higher self
Yum	Shiva	Green	Twelve Petals	Divine Love
Rum	Vishnu	Yellow	Ten Petals	Power instinct in man
Vum	Brahma	Orange	Six Petals	Pleasure instinct in man
Lum	Ganesh	Red	Four Petals	Survival instinct in man

Fulfilling desires is like pouring gasoline into a fire. The more they are gratified, the bigger they become.

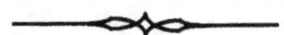

9

CONCENTRATION AND MEDITATION
(More details under Raja Yoga)

EXPLANATION
To keep the mind focused on any subject or object is called concentration. For example, mind can be focused on a candle flame or on the third eye. Concentration channels our energy and, therefore, our mind becomes clearer and sharper. A sharp mind is necessary for any accomplishment.

Sustained concentration leads into meditation. Meditation is done on any infinite aspect of God where the mind flows and expands. In meditation the knower, knowledge, and known become one. In this transcendental state one attains spiritual wisdom and guidance, and finds freedom from suffering.

PREPARATION
Sitting Position One should sit in lotus or any steady and comfortable position, keeping the spine erect. Then practice any yogic breathing to quiet the mind before practicing meditation.

Room The room should be quiet, comfortable, and pleasing. Use the same room and same spot; decorate the room with pictures of Saints or Guru.

Time Practice at the same time once or twice a day. Good times are early morning before starting the day and in the evening after completing your activities of the day.

General Practicing Yoga positions every day will help relax the body. Observe yogic dietary disciplines and follow yogic cleansing programs. (See Chapters 19 and 23.) Simplify your life style and be moderate in your sleep and activities. Read scriptures and associate with positive friends. These practices will help in mastering meditation and in reaching the depth of meditation.

METHODS

1. TRATAK

Tratak is an external concentration technique which uses the eyes. Eyes produce the strongest stimulus for the mind, but tratak converts this stimulus into a constructive concentration. It also strengthens eyes and eye muscles, increases control over nerve centers and the mind, and develops psychic powers.

Technique 1: Sit erect with the spine in a vertical position. Place a candle in front of you so the flame is slightly below eye level. Stare at the flame without blinking or straining your eyes. As soon as you feel tension in the eyes or they begin to water, close them and place your palms over them to relax the muscles.

Repeat the process, gradually increasing the duration of concentration. As you advance, try to visualize the candle flame between your eyebrows while your eyes are closed. Let the light expand to fill your body and continue expanding until the whole universe is covered by this light.

Technique 2: Concentrate on the tip of the nose instead of the candle flame. Follow the basic directions as stated above.

2. THIRD EYE

Concentration on the third eye is a very common technique of concentration. The third eye is located between the eyebrows. Our physical eyes see the material world, while the third eye sees through intuition. The third eye is also the location of the pineal gland. Focusing attention at this point naturally withdraws one's attention from the gross body, senses, and environment. Concentration on the third eye can also be combined with other concentration methods. In deep concentration our eyes are naturally drawn toward this center; conversely, by focusing our attention at this point we can produce deep concentration.

Technique: Sit in the meditative posture. Focus your closed or partially closed eyes at the point between the eyebrows without straining them. Do the palming whenever any tension is produced.

3. CONCENTRATION OF VARIOUS SENSES

One can concentrate on any of the five senses. One can withdraw the attention from particular sense objects or pick up one sound or sensation at the exclusion of all others. This is called Pratyahara and is described in Chapter 3, Raja Yoga.

4. SO HUM CONCENTRATION

This is a basic and time tested concentration technique. It is very easy and applicable for quiet meditation and can also be used as an active meditation while working during the day. In this technique the mind flows with the breath, which is easier than forcing the mind to a single point. Our mind is like a genie which is very obedient as long as you keep it busy. As soon as it is idle it destroys us. An idle mind is the devil's workshop. Keep the mind busy watching the breath whenever it is not occupied.

Technique: Sit in the meditation posture. Do deep breathing. Let the breathing become rhythmic and shallow. Observe your breath as a witness. Without trying to control anything, allow your mind to follow your breath until ultimately it identifies itself with it. You will experience your existence as a subtle breath connecting the gross body with the universe around it. The thought of being a physical body with weight disappears. The depth of concentration will increase with practice. Depth of concentration is more important than the length of concentration. Let all sounds and distractions remain in the background and avoid fighting them.

When you master this try the next step. Concentrate on the sound of inhalation which is So and the sound of exhalation which is Hum. After mastering the sound be aware of the meaning of So and Hum. So means that and Hum means I. Feel that I Am That. Feel that the absolute (That) is being united with your limited individual self (I) with the breath. Experience the after effect.

5. OM (AUM) MEDITATION

Om meditation is described in all the basic yogic scriptures. Om is the sound of creation. Chapter 11, Mantra Yoga, explains the theory of Om (Aum) and the meditation

technique. This method involves chanting Aum aloud and
mentally.

6. ASTRAL TRAVEL

We have three bodies: Physical, Astral, and
Causal. When we withdraw our awareness from our gross
body, we function at the astral body level. The astral body is
finer and subtler than our gross body and has freedom of travel
and movement.

Technique: This technique involves concentration
on various joints and centers as follows: the third eye, throat,
middle of chest, navel, pelvic center, all the joints of the arms and
legs, including wrists and ankles. The mental traveling starts at
the third eye, then to the throat, left arm, right arm, going down
through both legs, and returning back to the third eye.

Either sit in a meditation posture or lie down on
your back. Do deep breathing to quiet the mind. Let your mind
remain at one center for the duration of one breath in and one
breath out. Remain aware of one center at a time, then withdraw
your awareness from that general area. You will feel numbness
and feel as if that part of the body does not belong to you.
Progress in concentration downward and then return upward. If
you get deeply involved and go into deeper concentration, or
forget about concentrating on the points or forget where you
were, don't worry about it. This is normal.

The Astral Travel chart on the following page
indicates the direction of travel. Two techniques are effective:

1. Travel through the body from 1 to 33 taking
one inhalation and one exhalation at each point, experiencing
numbness and general relaxation in surrounding areas. At the
end, escape from the skull (34) into space and experience your
existence without size or shape, and become independent of the
body.

2. Travel from 1 to 29, then do one of the
following:

A. Travel up and down through the spine
being aware of one chakra at a time, taking one complete breath
(in and out) at each center.

B. Travel up the spine as you inhale and
down as you exhale.

ASTRAL TRAVEL

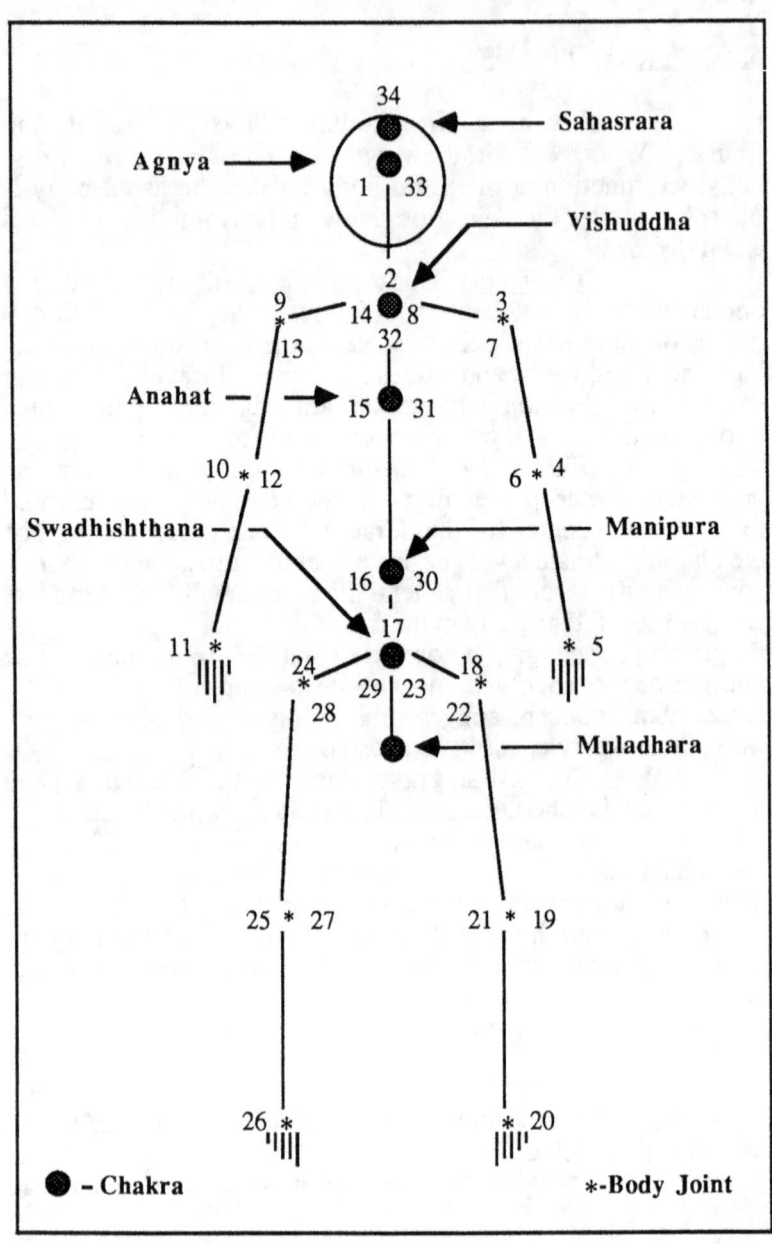

● – Chakra   *–Body Joint

7. GNANA YOGA MEDITATION

This technique involves the negative approach, I am not this (neti). One mentally repeats the mantra and feels that I am not this body, energy, mind, intellect, or ego. Then one uses the positive approach, Ahum Brahmasmi (I am Brahman). One feels union with the cosmic forces and dissolves his individual identity. This technique is explained in detail in Chapter 15, Gnana Yoga.

8. MANTRA YOGA MEDITATION

Technique 1: Mantras with vibrations. There are five Maha mantras (Universal mantras). They are described in Chapter 11, Mantra Yoga. Learn the pronunciation and tunes with a teacher. The technique and theory behind Mantra Yoga are described under the same chapter.

Technique 2: Bija mantras and mantras with affirmation. There are several seed mantras (Bija Mantras) which invoke energy by concentrating on them. There are also Vedic Mantras with positive affirmations, as in Thou Art That (Tat Twam Asi). All of these are explained in detail in Chapter 11, Mantra Yoga.

9. SELF ANALYSIS MEDITATION

One quiets the mind and inquires within: "Who am I?" One goes into deeper and deeper levels of meditation until he realizes that he is Atman (Self). This technique is explained in detail in Chapter 15, Gnana Yoga. This can also be applied as an active meditation technique.

10. PRANA AND SURRENDER TECHNIQUE

Technique 1: Surrender Yoga (Sharanagati Yoga) is described in Chapter 12.

Technique 2: Sit in a meditation position. Allow the body to be completely relaxed. During this technique the body is allowed full freedom to move. Withdraw the control of the mind from the body and let prana take over while the mind witnesses the entire process. Concentrate on the solar plexus (abdominal brain, located around the navel). Prana is stored at this center. Remain aware of prana at this location.

With each inhalation visualize prana rising from the solar plexus to the shoulders. With each exhalation, visualize prana flowing down to the arms, palms, and fingers. After a few rounds you will feel tingles in your fingers and palms. Palms and arms will be charged with prana and will start moving in different directions (this varies from person to person). Observe the process and do not try to control or stop it. Just be a witness and allow your body to experience this freedom. Initially try to keep your arms at shoulder level or move them consciously at an extremely slow speed until prana takes over the process.

At the end, consciously place your palms on your face and allow prana to transmit to your face, producing deep relaxation to this area and the rest of the body. Remain aware of the activities of prana throughout the body.

11. KUNDALINI MEDITATION

Technique 1: Sit in a meditation posture, observing your breath. Let your mind travel with your breath. Now let your attention travel up the spine with each inhalation and down with each exhalation. Prana is guided by one's awareness. Visualize and experience prana traveling the inner path of the spine (Shushumna), removing obstacles from its path and piercing the chakras within the spine. At the end sit quietly; feel that your entire spine is charged with energy rushing up and down.

Technique 2: This is a variation of Technique 1. Fold the tongue like a tube and extend it out. Sip the cool air as you breathe in. Then close the mouth and breathe out through the throat making a smooth sound. This is called Sitali Pranayama (cooling breathing). With inhalation visualize and feel a cool current traveling up the spine, and as you exhale travel down the spine feeling a warm current. Now experience the lowest center (muladhara) which represents Prakriti, uniting with the highest center (sahasrara) which represents Purusha.

Technique 3: Concentrate on one of the seven chakras located within the spine. Kundalini Yoga (See Chapter 8.) explains the location of each chakra and the corresponding Bija Mantra. Concentration invokes energy and helps awaken Kundalini.

Technique 4 Kriyas: There are several kriyas (techniques) which awaken Kundalini and produce meditative states of mind. Kriyas involve some breathing and visualization, and some movements. One should learn them under his Guru. (See Chapter 8 for details.)

12. EXPANSION

One may produce a quiet state of mind by any technique of breathing and meditation. One may visualize the divine light within the chamber of his heart and feel that light expanding and filling his entire body. Let expansion continue filling the entire room and completely covering everyone in the room. Allow it to expand in all directions until the town, country, world, and entire universe are filled with this light. Experience the oneness and lose your limited self in this meditation.

One may chant Aum and feel the expansion of his consciousness with the vibrations of the chant. Merge with these vibrations; become these universal vibrations. Feel the emotions of love, joy, and bliss generated within your heart. Feel the fountains of love flowing out in all directions until your entire body is saturated with love. Let it flow in all directions, reaching all the people in the room, until there is only love connecting you with the group. Expand until the whole universe around you is filled with love. Feel love within and without; feel that you are the universal love. This same technique can be applied to expand your individual joy and bliss with universal joy and bliss.

One can feel himself to be omnipresent, omnipotent, and omniscient. He can feel himself existing in everything and every being. One feels himself to be Brahman which is Sat (pure existence), Chit (pure consciousness), and Anand (pure bliss).

13. RECHARGING BREATHING

Practice recharging breathing as explained in Chapter 6, Breathing (Pranayama). Feel your body hto be porous like a sponge. Feel prana rushing through the pores of your skin. Imagine yourself floating in the ocean of prana, while your entire being dissolves and becomes one with the ocean.

14. MUDRAS

Mudras are gestures. Postures purify the body, while mudras purify the nadis (subtle nerve tubes) and help in awakening Kundalini. Some mudras resemble postures, but they are practiced differently than the postures. Mudras are guided by prana while the mind remains a witness. One should study mudras under the direct guidance of his Guru. (See Chapter 5 for details.)

15. DREAM EXPERIENCES-DEATH

These meditations help to break some basic attachments within ourselves. Meditation on death breaks the strong attachments to life, enjoyment, and the human body. One sees the transient nature of the world and the uncertainty of life. This will help develop intensity in your practice.

One can dwell on the dream experience and see life as a dream. Our emotions are short lasting. Life passes like waves. Being a witness, one transcends the experiences of life.

16. ACTIVE MEDITATION

Meditation and life style should not be separate things. Regular meditation affects our life. Living a proper and disciplined life helps our meditation. One can maintain harmony throughout the day. This is a form of active meditation. The Karma Yoga chapter explains how to perform our activities selflessly as a devotion to God so that our work becomes our worship. The chapter on Gnana Yoga explains the analysis and awareness techniques which can turn our activities into meditation.

One should chant the Guru Mantra <u>Om Namo Bhagavate Vasudevay (I surrender to the Divine),</u> until it becomes a constant meditation.

Worship God as a kind and forgiving Father, not as a punisher.

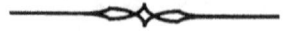

10

BHAKTI YOGA

The word Bhakti is derived from the Sanskrit root Bhaj, which means constant remembrance. Bhakti means constant remembrance of God. According to Saint Narada, "Bhakti is intense love for God." When one becomes intoxicated by this love, one loves all, hates none, and is satisfied. Gnana Yogi Shankara describes Bhakti as the relentless search after one's Self and, even on the path of Gnana Yoga, Bhakti is required. Ramanuja defines deep meditation as a form of Bhakti. Like the flow of oil from one container to another, the practicing Bhakta's mind flows on the thoughts of his beloved deity like the flowing of oil.

Love is God. From love the world is created, in love it exists, and in love it returns. Love is the law of life. A mother develops love for her newborn child and brings up the child with tender care. All animals have instinctive love for their offspring. Love is living. Love is the goal of life. Without love life is a burden. Even criminals experience love in their hearts for some people and in certain situations. Directing this love towards God is the goal of Bhakti Yoga.

The love most people know is transitory love for material possessions, friends, and relatives. This love only brings temporary happiness because all objects of the world are temporary, subject to change and decay. They are bound by the Law of Karma (cause and effect), existing in time and space. When these objects are destroyed, one feels sorrow. Love for God, however, is permanent. It brings joy in the beginning, middle, and at the end. Bhakti Yoga is the technique of transforming our limited love into supreme love for God. Human life is filled with emotions, love being a common emotion for all. Its seat is in the heart. Emotions can drain our energy but when they are changed into love, they bring joy and happiness. Love conquers the world. All emotions, such as hate and anger, can be controlled through love. Bhakti Yoga techniques convert negative destructive emotions into constructive love for God.

Human love is conditional and possessive while love for God is unconditional. We hold onto loved ones, become attached to them, or may even, in some instances, become jealous of them. If we offer love and there is no positive response, we become disturbed, which in turn produces anxiety. Loving God is unconditional. We love for the sake of loving with no strings attached. As our consciousness expands our ego dissolves and we experience bliss all the time.

Love is a spontaneous experience. There are no words to describe it. Human love is selfish and there is confusion between love and thoughts of love. While thinking and talking about love, we are distracted from the experience itself. When love is experienced, doubts disappear. Unnecessary talk about love is an indication of the lack of love.

Experience of love is the experience of God because love is God. Human love is emotional and springs from the mind. In the true experience of love, mind and emotions disappear. Bhakti is a spontaneous love. Flowers emit fragrance without effort, and the sun shines without effort. In the same way, the Bhakta's heart longs for God. In order to experience such a spontaneous love, we must first purify ourselves with the practice of Yamas and Niyamas. (See Chapter 3, Raja Yoga.)

God is our Mother, we are her children. For a mother's attention a child may cry and nag or make playful gestures. Austere disciplines of other branches of Yoga are like a nagging child, while Bhakti Yoga is a playing child. The Bhakti Yogi attracts God with his love. It is easier to attract God with love than with nagging .

In other branches of Yoga the techniques are used to attain liberation. In Bhakti Yoga Bhakti is the means and Bhakti is the end. We do not have to struggle for liberation. Serving God with Bhakti is liberation. God tries to tempt yogis with siddhis (yogic supernatural powers), as a mother tries to keep her child busy by providing a variety of toys. A Bhakti Yogi, however, wants God his Mother, instead of siddhis (toys). In the ninth chapter of the Gita, Shri Krishna explains, "The worshipers of Gods go to the Gods; worshipers of the spirits go to the spirit, and the worshipers of me come to me. Those persons who think only of me, I look after their maintenance and welfare."

With Bhakti, God can be pleased very easily. Krishna says, "Even if a Bhakta offers me a leaf, a flower, fruit, or water, with a pure mind, I accept it." Love and devotion are the greatest offerings one can make to please the Lord. The material alms are not important. The greatest sacrifice we can make to please the Lord is to sacrifice our ego and surrender to Him with humility. Krishna says, "Whatever you do, or eat, or sacrifice, whatever austerity you perform, offer unto me."

Bhakti produces Satvik faith. This faith is of a dynamic nature and allows one to use his intellect and rational faculties. It is based upon experience. A lower form of faith is rigid, lacks understanding and compassion for living beings. It is based upon dogma and theory. This blind faith is the product of ignorance and is called Tamasik faith. People with Tamasik faith obtain enlightenment eventually, whereas those without faith have no direction or peace of mind.

The major textbooks of Bhakti Yoga are:

1. **Bhakti Rasamrita Sindhu** Written by a disciple of Chaitanya Mahaprabhu, a great Bhakti Yogi of about 500 years ago.

2. **Narada Bhakti Sutras** Written by unknown authors and named after a mythological Bhakti Yogi Saint Narada.

3. **Bhagavad Gita** Chapter 12 is dedicated to Bhakti Yoga. Many other chapters, however, also bring out the glories of Bhakti.

There are two kinds of Bhakti: Gauni (preparatory) and Para (supreme). Gauni Bhakti is based upon reason and motive, and one worships God for some sort of gain. This is a lower form of Bhakti. Para Bhakti is Bhakti with supreme love, without any selfish motivation. Gauni Bhakti eventually ripens into Para Bhakti. Gauni Bhakti is of three kinds: Tamasik, Rajasik, and Satvik.

Tamasik Bhakti is deluded and blind and manifests as violence and jealousy. God is appealed to for revenge of the worshiper's enemies. Rajasik Bhakti is egotistic and passionate, hence wealth, fame, and pleasures are sought. Satvik Bhakti is pure Bhakti. The devotee seeks enlightenment, adores and surrenders to God, and considers Bhakti as his duty.

Four kinds of Bhaktas pray to God.

1. ARTRA, or distressed and suffering. One who feels completely rejected in all situations turns to God. This Bhakti is temporary. God is easily forgotten as soon as this apparent rejection turns to acceptance or when suffering ends.

2. ARTHARTHI, or mendicant. This Bhakta is hungry for prosperity. He worships God to acquire wealth and power.
3. JIGNASU, or inquiring. God is searched for out of curiosity.
4. GNANI, or the man of wisdom. He worships with complete understanding without any selfish motives and is not distracted from his Bhakti. He has the foundation for Bhakti. Krishna says, "Out of these four kinds of seekers, the man of wisdom is the best. He is constantly established in identity with me and is possessed with exclusive devotion. I am extremely dear to the wise man and he is extremely dear to me. Out of thousands of men, few struggle for perfection. Out of those perhaps only one becomes perfect and attains me in reality."

Even if one prays for selfish ends, he will attain them as long as he is praying sincerely. Men of wisdom ask for no selfish reward. They ask for the lotus feet of the Lord so that they may serve him constantly. Prayers that bring results are the prayers that come from the depth of the heart. These prayers are not performed for show but are done privately.

A devotee cries in his prayers. Many people shed tears because of their problems, but very few people pray and cry because they feel separated from God. We cannot pray with our whole heart as long as we are caught up in pleasures of the world.

To find God one needs intense love for Him. A mother has great attachment to her newborn, a miser is attached to his wealth, and there is a strong bond of love between a newlywed bride and groom. If one's intensity in his love for God exceeds the combined love of the above situations, one finds God.

A Guru taught a lesson to explain the intensity of Bhakti to his disciple by taking him to a lake and holding his head under water. The disciple was puzzled at the crazy act of his Guru. The Guru explained that, when you were pushed under the water, you were thinking of a gasp of air and nothing else. In the same way, if you yearn for God to the exclusion of all other desires, you will attain God.

Gauni Bhakti involves rituals, such as austerities, fasting, chanting, worshiping your chosen deity, singing bhajans (devotional songs), doing Arti, donating to charities, and reading scriptures. All of these disciplines are preparatory Bhakti. They purify the mind and heart, and invoke love and devotion in the heart of a devotee. Eventually, when the rituals become unnecessary and one worships the formless universal God, Bhakti has grown into Para Bhakti. God is then seen as manifested in all living beings. These two kinds of Bhakti are explained in the 12th chapter of the Gita.

Arjuna asks Krishna, "Out of two kinds of Bhaktas, those who worship the personal God and those who worship the impersonal God, who are the better Bhaktas?" Krishna says, "Those who worship the unmanifest, all pervading, changeless and eternal, by controlling their senses, are even minded and devoted to the good of all beings, attain to me alone, but their path is harder. While those who renounce all actions to me, are attached to me, worship me in personal form with unswerving devotion through meditation, I save them quickly. This is an easier path for the embodied soul."

Worship of personal deities is easy for the average person. It is easier to focus on a symbol or personal God and His attributes than to focus on an impersonal God. A devotee uses his body and senses while living in the world of relativity. The eyes are used for seeing his personal God, the mouth for singing his glories; the ears are used to hear of his glories, the hands for serving him and playing instruments, and the legs are used for dancing in his ecstasy. This is an easy approach for the average person.

We can worship God with different Bhavas (modes of love). We can worship God as his servant (Dasya Bhava), a friend (Sakha Bhava), as parents (Vatsalya Bhava), as our own self (Shanta Bhava), or as a bride of God (Madhura Bhava). Traditional practice is to consider God as a beloved. One becomes a female lover of God, as a Gopi.

HOW TO DEVELOP BHAKTI

There are nine practices used for developing Bhakti. They are called Navadha Bhakti.

1. SHRAVANA (Hearing the stories of God) One listens to the stories of the scriptures from the Ramayana, Mahabarata, and Bhagavatam, where the incarnations of Rama and Krishna performed Lilas (divine plays). This purifies the mind and the heart. One may listen to the Vedas and Upanishads. They are Srutis. One may listen to the life stories of the saints. One should listen to the words of his Guru. After listening carefully, he should do Manana (reflecting) and then Nididhyas (meditating). These provide constant inspiration.

2. KIRTAN (Singing and chanting the holy names of God) Sing His glories, adore Him, sing Mahamantras (accompanied by instruments) with love in your heart, and dance. Write devotional songs (Bhajans) and get involved in different Bhavas (divine moods of ecstasy). In Kali Yuga (the present age), Kirtana is highly recommended. It is easy, effective, does not require knowledge of scriptures nor does it require severe austerities.

3. SMARANA (Remembering one's deity) By remembering His glories, His teachings and incidents from the scriptures which are inspirational, one's Bhakti increases. Remembering different Bhaktas and their life stories, how they maintained their faith in critical test situations, remembering one's own Guru and his teachings, the memories of time spent with Guru, and the blissful experiences of meditation - all of these increase Bhakti. You should chant the Guru Mantra when your mind is not occupied. Meditate on the image of God.

4. PADA SEVA (Serving the Lord and waiting upon Him) In a ritualistic worship one establishes an altar and sets up an image, picture, or statue of his beloved deity. He then devotes his full attention as if God were present in human form. The devotee wakes up God, bathes Him, feeds Him, clothes Him, and puts Him to sleep with Bhava (deep feelings). Flowers and fruits are presented as prasad (offerings). This invokes unconditional love in the heart of the Bhakta. The Guru is considered as his living God. Since the Guru is physically present, he serves him with love. Guru Seva and spending time in his presence are part of his routine practice. Ultimately this service is expanded to elders, needy, sick, and animals. All living beings are served, seeing the living God in them.

5. ARCHANAM (Worship) One worships his idol by ritualistic means as explained in the scriptures. There are sixteen types of Poojas (worship). They involve symbolic offerings of flowers, fruits, Arti (fire ceremony). Internal worship means constant remembrance and chanting His name. One establishes the image of his idol in his heart and worships him constantly while performing various duties during the day.

6. VANDANAM (Salutation) The devotee prostrates in front of the idol. The highest prostration is Shastang dundavat namaskar (when the six parts of the body are touching the floor, with arms and legs stretched out straight, lying on the stomach). He prostrates in front of his Guru. Real prostration is humility. He demonstrates respect to the Guru, Saints, elders, and all beings by bowing down and giving greetings (Jai Bhagwan).

7. DASYA (Servantship to God) The greatest joy is in serving God. When God asks his devotees what boons they desire, they always ask for servantship to Him.

8. SAKHYA (Friendship with God) Many devotees worship Him as a friend. Arjuna of the Gita worshiped Krishna as a friend.

9. ATMA NIVEDANA (Self surrender) One surrenders to God completely. He performs his duties and leaves the results to the Lord. The highest surrender is giving up one's own ego.

On the path of Yoga one needs a Guru. A Guru is a spiritual teacher and guide. He has tread the path and guides his disciple on the path. The Guru has purity of heart and the spiritual strength to help his disciple. He is a man of vision. A blind man cannot lead another blind man. A disciple should follow his Guru to gain spiritual strength.

Dispassion and non-attachment help one in Bhakti. Attachment to worldly mundane matters takes attention away from God. Yama and Niyamas should be practiced to purify the consciousness. One should renounce the six vices which lead to degradation, which are considered the six enemies of humans. They are: 1. Kama (lust), 2. Krodha (anger), 3. Matsara (jealousy and hate), 4. Lobha (greed), 5. Mada (vanity), and 6. Moha (infatuation).

Satsang (company of the saints) is recommended for maintaining constant awareness of the goal. One can have satsang of scriptures and writings of saints and can keep friends with higher (purer) interests in life. Whenever the mind is not occupied, chant the Guru Mantra for satsang.

Other phases of life cannot be avoided. It is always helpful to practice Hatha Yoga regularly so the body feels harmonious with the mind. Also practice Karma Yoga (selfless service) and Gnana Yoga (constant awareness). Practice all branches of Yoga in proper proportion. Gnana and Bhakti are the two wings while Karma and Raja Yoga form the rudder which controls the direction on the path.

All paths of Yoga meet at the same goal eventually. Bhakti Yoga, however, is the easiest path for the average person in society. Most religions of the world are following the Bhakti Yoga path. It is ideal for most people.

See the spark of God in all living creatures, even though they manifest different pleasant or unpleasant qualities. This is how we can accept and love them as they are and learn something from them. Each person has some deeper wisdom and unique talent. By not judging people we communicate and learn from them.

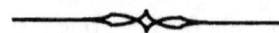

Learn to trust your innerself. Masses of people without inner awakening follow the crowd like sheep with head down and without long range vision. A brave person with inner conviction travels alone and invents new trails. Learn to trust what you see and feel in the weather instead of just believing the forecast. Learn to tune into people instead of accepting prejudices and opinions you may have heard about them. Judgment interferes with truth and experience.

If you want to bathe in the ocean, jump in now. Don't wait for the waves to subside. If you want to start something worthwhile, start now. Disturbing waves never stop in life.

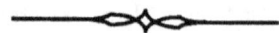

11

MANTRA YOGA

The goal of Yoga is unity with the higher self. In Mantra Yoga this goal is reached by repetition of certain sounds and invocations which were perceived by great Rishis during their deep meditation. "MANANAT TRAYATE ITI MANTRAH" means constant repetition of the mantra protects one from the ocean of Maya (illusion). Some invocations have meaning or contain spiritual vibrations, while other mantras are holy names and praises of the divine God. These produce love and devotion in the heart of the practitioner, thus resembling Bhakti Yoga.

The goal of Yoga is to attain liberation. Different paths were recommended for different Yugas (Ages) to fulfill this aim in the most applicable way. In Satya Yuga (the Age of Purity) meditation was recommended. In Treta Yuga (the Age of the loss of Truth) sacrifices were recommended. In Dwapar Yuga (the Age of the loss of Compassion and Truth) worship and prayers were recommended. Our present age is Kali Yuga (the Dark Age) where evil forces and immorality prevail, Mantra Yoga is highly recommended.

KALI YUGE KEVAL NAMA ADHARA. In Kali Yuga the holy name of the divine God is like a boat which, when utilized, saves man and helps him cross the ocean of Maya to attain Self-realization.

Bhakti Sutras say that sweeter than all sweets, more auspicious than good things and purer than pure things is the name of God. The name of God is a tool for conquering the mind.

NAMA (Name) and RUPA (Form) are inseparable. In our imaginations the word *summer* produces heat and the word *winter* produces cold. In the same way, chanting the names of God produces the image of God and reminds us of Him and His glories. Most people feel trapped by problems, tension, and worries of all kinds. Chanting the holy name removes these worries and produces peace of mind.

Some people can benefit more from one mantra than another because mantras have different effects on different people. An evolved Guru can determine which mantra would be best for a disciple. Guru determines this by studying a disciple for many years after which the mantra is given with proper initiation (Diksha). The power of the mantra increases after the initiation, for one becomes united with the power of a chain of Gurus who are behind the mantra. After receiving the Guru Mantra one does not need to chant a variety of mantras. If one chants other mantras, he still maintains the devotion to the Guru Mantra.

There are six aspects of each mantra:

1. RISHI: A self-realized Rishi (Yogi) who perceived the mantra in deep meditation and gave it to the world. Mantras are universal and have no language barrier.

2. METRE: This governs the inflection of the voice.

3. DEVATA: Personal God. He is the presiding deity of the mantra and is the informing power.

4. BIJA: Seed. This is a significant basic word or letter which gives special power to the mantra. As a tree is hidden in a seed, so the energy of a mantra is hidden in the Bija. A tree grows from a seed by nourishing it. In the same way, by repeating the mantra the Bija is nourished and energy is generated.

5. SHAKTI: Energy. All mantras have potency which is released by repetition. This potency takes a man to the Devata (God) of the mantra.

6. KILAKA: This is the pillar which supports the entire mantra. It fastens the mantra together. This bond is removed by constant repetition.

BENEFITS

Mantras have a relaxing effect, producing deep relaxation to those who chant them and also to those who listen to them. Mantras are used in curing many diseases and in solving other problems. They produce deep relaxation in the subconscious mind where the roots of our problems, such as diseases, are hidden. The vibrations of the mantra penetrate the physical and astral bodies of the practitioner and fill the cells with satva (purity), which is the best medicine for all problems.

In mantra chanting the body and senses are forgotten and one becomes absorbed in the joy of the Divine. Meditation is used for transcending the lower nature of the body and mind. Mantra chanting helps quiet the mind and leads one into meditation. Those who cannot control the restless mind through other techniques can easily tame it through mantra chanting. Our social structure and life style promote the overuse of our mind, logic, etc. and our heart center is inactive. Mantra chanting opens our heart center, balances our personality, and removes stress. It is an effective meditation technique for persons with an active and restless mind.

Mantra chanting purifies and strengthens the spiritual samskaras. These are hidden impressions in the subconscious mind. Good and bad samskaras (karmas) are produced by thought, word, and deed. A man becomes what he thinks. The character of a man is built by continuous good thoughts. Mantras are positive affirmations which produce strong impressions and transform a person. Also, they bring negative samskaras to the surface and burn them to ashes, speeding spiritual evolution.

Mantra purifies the heart, develops love towards all, brings peace of mind, and helps awaken Kundalini. The devotee feels the presence of the Divine protecting him at all times. Mantra is a protective shield against negative and disturbing forces such as worry, fear, loneliness, and restlessness.

Mantra affects the brain wave pattern, producing alpha brain waves. This is a creative state of mind and develops the creative forces lying dormant within us. Ultimately, it reveals true knowledge of the Self.

Mantra is a spiritual soap which removes the dirt of the mind. Yoga describes six mental enemies of man called SHAD RIPU. They are: 1. KAMA, 2. KRODHA, 3. LOBHA, 4. MADA, 5. MOHA, and 6. MATSARA. These are desires, anger, greed, wrong pride, passion, and hatred. Mantra also changes Rajas (restlessness) and Tamas (dullness) into Satva (purity), along with controlling the six enemies.

Mantra chanting fulfills four PURUSHARTHAS (aims in life), which are: 1. Dharma (spiritual happiness), 2. Artha (material happiness), 3. Kama (sensual happiness), and 4. Moksha (liberation).

Sounds and images have a very close relationship. Certain sounds produce certain images. The mantra of Krishna produces the image of Krishna; the mantra of Shiva produces the image of Lord Shiva. Mantra chanting invokes the deity of the mantra because the deity and the mantra are one and the same. One attracts the divine qualities of the deity by chanting his mantra. Divinity flows from the deity to his practitioner, and ultimately the practitioner becomes the deity whom he worships. The mind becomes what it thinks of constantly.

The power of the mantra cannot be understood by intellectual thinking but only through practice. Water does not quench our thirst by thinking about it, we must drink it. One should experiment by keeping the mind open and receptive in order to verify the power of mantras. After the experience doubts are dispelled. Just as fire has the property to burn those who touch it even if they don't know about it, in the same way mantra chanting and listening dispel ignorance and give inner peace.

Many great masters have chanted these mantras. The power of the mantra builds over the years. Those who chant the mantra derive the help and power from these great masters of the past.

Our body is a microcosm. All the Gods and Goddesses are within our body. For example, Lord Vishnu (the Sustainer) resides in the navel. As Vishnu sustains the microcosm so the navel region (the solar plexus) sustains the life force and activities of the body. Invoking Lord Vishnu means invoking the hidden energy within the body.

Man does not live by bread alone. Mantra chanting is spiritual food for Yoga practitioners.

DIFFERENT KINDS OF MANTRAS

A. MANTRA WITH VIBRATIONS

There are some mantras which have no external meaning. Usually they are the holy names of God. For example, Maha mantras produce vibrations when they are chanted, which affect the nervous system of the person chanting and also of those listening. Studies have shown that chanting these mantras produces alpha brain waves which bring about a state of deep relaxation and meditation.

These mantras are definite invocations involving a specific kind of breathing while chanting them. This breathing is a type of pranayama which has a cleansing and purifying effect on the body and mind. Rhythmic sound is called music and without rhythm, sound becomes noise. Rhythm relaxes the nerves, while noise disturbs the nerves. Mantras are rhythmic sound vibrations. The clapping of hands and playing of musical instruments are used along with chanting, which help attune the mind to the rhythm.

Mantras with vibrations are best and most effective when practiced in a group with instruments and clapping. There are definite tunes to these mantras, yet one may use any suitable tune in chanting them. In deep meditation one lets himself go; the chanting becomes automatic and new melodious tunes are produced. This happens when one's Vishuddha Chakra opens up. It is called ANAHAT NADA which means automatic chanting. Om, Hari Om, and Rama mantras are commonly used in Anahat Nada.

B. MANTRAS WITH MEANING (Affirmations)

These are short mantras with definite meaning and positive affirmations; e.g., Ahum Brahmasmi (I am Brahman). They are ideal for mental japas and can be practiced while working, eating, or driving a car.

While chanting these mantras, one should dwell on the meaning. The meaning penetrates the conscious mind and then reaches the subconscious level, and ultimately reaches the supreme mind where it carves new impressions, develops positive and elevating samskaras, and removes deep-rooted negative impressions. Our inner mind is the root cause of many physical and psychological diseases, which can be removed by positive affirmations.

Man is what he thinks. Depending upon the mantra, chanting attracts the right people and environment so that ultimately, all affirmations are materialized. If one repeats the mantras of surrender, he feels the presence and protection of the Divine Being guiding him and providing help when needed. When one chants So Hum (I am That) mantra he feels the divinity within and is able to throw off the ignorance of the lower self (body, mind, emotions, etc.), and he transcends the duality created by the mind. When one repeats the mantra of a particular deity, he attracts the divine qualities of that deity and eventually becomes the deity himself.

Mantra chanting is not hypnotic suggestion. Hypnotic suggestion sets limits to our potential by saying "I am capable of doing this or that." Mantra affirmations are the process of dehypnotism. We have hypnotized ourselves over the years of repeated incarnations and are in bondage to the body, mind, time, and space. Mantra affirmations declare that I am Brahman - the pure being - SAT, CHIT, and ANAND (pure existence, knowledge, and bliss).

By repeating the mantra mentally over a long period of time, it becomes automatic chanting called Ajapa Japa. Mantra chanting goes on with each breath. (We take about 21,600 breaths during a day.) Ajapa Japa continues while sleeping, dreaming, working, and thinking. Part of the mind chants the mantra constantly which protects and guides the practitioner. After prolonged practice of Ajapa Japa one attains MANTRA SIDDHI or mastery of the mantra. A person who has this Mantra Siddhi can fulfill any wish just by uttering the mantra once. Evolved masters never misuse this mantra power. Many examples have been seen in India where people were healed by Mantra Siddha masters just by their uttering the mantra once.

Even if one does not become a Mantra Siddha, the power of the mantra accumulates. This accumulated power comes to the aid of the practitioner in times of distress.

C. SATVIK, RAJASIK, and TAMASIK MANTRAS

1. Satvik mantras are used to attain the highest goal of purification and Self-realization.

2. Rajasik mantras are used for the purposes of gaining wealth, power, and to satisfy lower desires.

3. Tamasik mantras are used for the control of evil spirits, hurting others and taking revenge.

Tamasik mantras give results very fast. Results of Rajasik mantras take a long time, while Satvik mantras take the longest length of time to produce results. All mantras given in this book are Satvik mantras.

D. SAGUNA and NIRGUNA MANTRAS

Brahman (the supreme being) is without form and is all pervading but due to the devotion of his Bhakta (devotee) he takes different forms, just as water turns to ice and assumes different forms. The Brahma without form is called Nirguna Brahman, and the Brahman with form is called Saguna Brahman. The mantra used for personal God or Saguna Brahman is called Saguna mantra, and the mantra used for impersonal or Nirguna Brahman is called Nirguna mantra. The worship of personal gods like Krishna, Rama, Buddha, and Christ is easy for the average person. Then, once the mind is focused, it becomes easy to attain the knowledge of Nirguna Brahman which exists within and without.

Saguna mantras are praises and appeals to the deities. These mantras involve Bhakti (devotion) and many rituals for pleasing the personal God. For example, the mantra OM NAMAH SHIVAYA is for pleasing Lord Shiva.

Saguna Mantra
(Worship of a particular deity)

OM SHRI KRISHNAY NAMAH
I worship Lord Krishna

OM SHRI RAMAY NAMAH
I worship Lord Rama

OM SHRI MAHA GANAPATAYE NAMAH
I worship Lord Ganapati

OM SHRI HANUMATE NAMAH
I worship Lord Hanuman

SRI KRISHNAH SHARANAM MAMA
Lord Krishna is my shelter

OM SHRI SARASWATYAI NAMAH
I worship Goddess Saraswati
(Goddess of Wisdom and Learning)

OM SHRI MAHALAXMYAI NAMAH
I worship Goddess Lakshmi
(Goddess of Prosperity)

OM NAMO BHAGAVATE VASUDEVAY
I worship Lord Vasudeva

OM NAMAH SHIVAY

I worship Lord Shiva. Panchakshara Mantra (five letters). OM is Bija, Namah is Shakti, Shivay is Kilakam.

OM NAMO NARAYANAYA

I worship Lord Narayana. Eight lettered mantra. Om is Bija, Narayana is Rishi, Narayana is Devata.

Nirguna mantras are affirmations like That is I, I am Brahman, etc. One affirms that he is created in the image of God and that God exists in everything.

E. JAPA, DHOONA, and BHAJANA

Constant repetition of mantra is called Japa. Krishna says in the Gita: Yagnanam Japa Yagnosmi, which means "Among the Yagnas (sacrifices) I am Japa." The greatest sacrifice one can make to please the Lord is to utter his name. The Lord likes to hear his name and runs to his devotee to help when his name is chanted. Japa leads one into meditation.

There are three kinds of Japas: Vaikhari or audible, Upamshu or whisper, and Pashyanti or mental and ethereal. Mental chanting is more powerful than audible chanting. The chanter ultimately reaches Para State or the transcendental state of sound. This potential or causal state of sound is beyond the barriers of language.

When chanting is done in rhythm at a faster speed with instruments and clapping it is called Dhoona; e.g., Rama Dhoona. Bhajans are the inspirational poems and devotional songs describing the glories of God. Bhajans help persons evolve by elevating their consciousness. Many were written by saints and holy men in their meditations.

HOW TO CHANT MANTRAS AND JAPAS

After taking a shower or washing hands and feet, put on fresh clothes and sit in a steady position on a woolen blanket to conserve body energy and prevent penetration of lower earthly vibrations. Practice in a definite place and at a regular time for maximum benefits. Increase the time for japa regularly and do not allow any gap in the practice. Before starting japa, do some pranayama followed by a prayer. This helps quiet the mind. Pronounce the mantra correctly, keeping the mind alert and avoiding distractions and sleepiness. Best results are obtained by observing the Yogic disciplines of Yamas and Niyamas during the course of Mantra Upasana (spiritual practice). Celibacy is highly recommended during Mantra Upasana.

Concentrate and dwell on the meaning of the mantra. Mantra chanted with concentration is superior to mechanical chanting. Do not rush when you are finished chanting. Remain attuned to the vibrations and after effects.

Chanting the mantra with Bhava (feeling and emotion) becomes Bhakti Yoga. Bhakti means earnest longing. The devotee longs to see God, like a lover longs to see his beloved. Those who worship Saguna Brahman should concentrate on the picture of the deity, feeling that the deity is sending him mercy and love. Surrender your body, mind, and ego at the feet of the deity. Visualize the image of the deity with closed eyes and feel that your deity is listening to you and protecting you. Those who worship Nirguna Brahman should visualize divine light in the chamber of the heart from where they are witnessing everything.

Tears are shed for worldly things and for petty problems. If one sheds even a few tears in the longing and love for God, God comes running to him.

In worshiping, one should keep the feeling of Dasya Bhava (being a servant of God), Putra Bhava (being a son of God), Gopi Bhava (being a female love of God), or Sakha Bhava (being a friend of God). With these feelings in the heart, one reaches Bhava Samadhi or union with God. This samadhi is easier to attain than the samadhi attained by the severe disciplines of Raja Yoga. In the practice of severe disciplines one nags God for liberation, whereas in Bhakti Yoga the devotee pleases God with Prem, or love, and God comes running.

During group chanting one may use Vaikhari Japa, which is chanting aloud with instruments and clapping. Chanters may also dance in the ecstasy of divine joy. While chanting alone, chant slower and slower until it becomes a whisper and ultimately becomes mental. Mental chanting is far superior to audible chanting.

Mantra chanting may be done while doing Karma Yoga. An idle mind is the devil's workshop. The mind has a natural tendency to worry, think, daydream, and drain energy. Mantra chanting brings the mind under control and, if performed while doing other activities, becomes active meditation. Work becomes meditation and worship to God. Chanting mentally with each breath becomes Ajapa Japa (automatic chanting), and one remains in the higher plane of awareness and consciousness while engaged in activities of a lower level.

A Bhakta may practice writing a certain number of mantras every day. Mantra writing is helpful in concentration because it centers a wandering mind. This is called Likhit Mantra or written mantra. Mental chanting leads one to meditation. People with restless and disturbed minds find it hard to quiet the mind and cannot meditate. Therefore mantra chanting is a very helpful method for them.

You may chant one mantra or several in combination. Those who have received the Guru Mantra should primarily do Japas of the Guru Mantra and chant all others when with a group.

The power and benefits of Mantra and Japa can be realized only through practice and cannot be understood intellectually.

USE OF MALA (ROSARY) FOR JAPA

A mala is useful in developing a disciplined practice. Its use brings alertness when the mind begins to drift or feels sleepy. The mala releases nervous energy by using the fingers which increases concentration during prolonged Japa. The mala reminds one of God and of higher goals in life. The mala is a rosary consisting of 108 beads and a large bead called Meru (holy mountain). The beads are made of the Tulasi plant or Rudraksha. Tulasi has therapeutic value. Wearing it around the neck produces a positive influence on the heart.

Use the right hand for turning the mala. Let it hang on the ring finger, supported with the thumb. Turn one bead with each chant of the mantra using the middle finger. Do not cross the Meru. When you come to the Meru, reverse the mala and continue. Do a definite number of malas every day.

BIJA MANTRA AND OM CHANTING

Bija means seed. The seed of a tree has the potential of becoming a tree if the proper environment is provided. Bija mantra is the basic and vital part of each mantra. Constant chanting of the mantra opens up the hidden power of this seed. Bija mantra usually contains a single syllable or sometimes several syllables. Each Bija mantra represents a Devata (deity) and has a deep meaning which is revealed by experience. This meaning is subtle and mystical.

Our body is a microcosm and all the Devatas reside within it. When one invokes a certain Devata, he opens up a certain potential within his consciousness. Our spine is called Meru Dunda. As Mount Meru supports the whole universe (according to Hindu scriptures) so our spine supports the micro universe within our body. The chakras (wheels or centers) exist in the inner subtle region of the spine and are pierced as one evolves spiritually. Each chakra has a definite location, Devata, and Bija mantra. (See Chapter 8 for details.) By concentration on these centers and its Bija mantra, the corresponding deity is invoked.

The best Bija mantra for you can be determined by an evolved Guru or by an expert astrologer. OM is the most powerful of all Bija mantras.

OM or A U M

The real OM sound is called Amatra or immeasurable sound, which is heard in deep meditation. "In the beginning was the word and the word was with God, and the word was God." says Saint John in the new testament of the Bible. "In the beginning was Prajapati with whom was the word, and the word was supreme Brahman" according to the Vedas. Supreme Brahman is represented by OM. "Among the words, I am Pranav (OM)," says Lord Krishna in the Gita.

Sounds produce feelings and images. As the word *snow* produces a chill in our imagination, in the same way the word OM produces the image of God and reminds us of God. In different languages there are different invocations to represent God. OM represents God without barriers of language or time.

AUM represents the entire phenomena of sound production. A is the root sound of most languages. It can be pronounced without the use of the palate or tongue. U rolls from the beginning to the end of the sounding board. M is the ending sound which is pronounced with closed lips. AUM altogether covers the entire range of sounds that can ever be pronounced and is represented by a single lettered symbol as shown on page 109.

Nirguna Brahman (Impersonal God) is represented by the trinity of Gods: Brahma the Creator, Vishnu the Sustainer, and Shiva the Transformer. The entire universe begins in Brahman, is sustained in Brahman, and dissolves in Brahman, but Brahman remains unchanged. A represents Brahma, U represents Vishnu, and M represents Shiva, and the entire symbol of AUM, pronounced OM, represents Para Brahma which includes all the forces of nature and transcends them all.

Newton's disk of seven colors which, when spun at high speed, appears white. In the same way, when all the sounds of the universe combine, the AUM sound is heard.

The Latin word omni and the Sanskrit AUM are derived from the same root. Both mean the Omnipresent, Omnipotent, and Omniscient nature of God. Gita uses the word Pranav to represent AUM. The root NU means praise. The best prayer to God can be offered by chanting AUM.

A represents Jagrat or waking state, U represents Swapna or dream state, and M represents Susupta or dreamless sleep state. The symbol of AUM represents Turiya, or Samadhi, and includes and transcends all states of consciousness. A is the past, U is the present, and M is the future. AUM is the creator who transcends time. A is Satva or purity, U is Rajas or activity, and M is Tamas or inertia. AUM is Gunatit, beyond guna.

AUM chanting produces definite vibrations which are soothing, relaxing, and healing for those who chant or listen. It leads the mind into deep meditation by the production of alpha brain waves. Consciousness expands and one feels harmony and union with nature and other living beings.

HOW TO CHANT OM OR AUM

Take a deep breath and visualize the sound coming from the navel. A sound comes from the depth, U sound rolls through the sounding board, and M sound comes with closed lips until one is out of breath. The entire chant is done in one breath without a break. While chanting, feel the vibrations in the entire body, the expansion of your consciousness, and the merging with nature until you experience omnipresence. In group chanting, continue chanting OM with a new deep breath each time, and let your sound merge with the sound vibrations of the group. Continue for a few minutes. At the conclusion of chanting, remain at ease and feel the after effect and vibrations. Slowly open your eyes while remaining in this calm state.

MENTAL OM CHANTING

Close your ears with your thumbs and place your fingers over the eyes. Listen to all the sounds in the inner ear while keeping the closed eyes focused on the Agnya Chakra (between the eyebrows). Transcend the grosser sounds and try to listen to the subtle sounds until a continuous OM sound is heard. Tune up the mind to this sound while keeping the ears open. This is a very effective technique of meditation.

GURU MANTRA

The Guru Mantra is given by a Guru to a disciple when the disciple is initiated into Yoga. Swami Shri Kripalvanandji is my Guru. The following mantra is for those who follow my teachings.

OM NAMO BHAGAVATE VASUDEVAY
I surrender to the Divine

This mantra is the Mantra of Surrender. It is open to all regardless of culture or nationality but becomes more effective after initiation. It can be chanted in a group with clapping and instruments or it can be chanted mentally.

This mantra becomes more effective when one is initiated and links up to the chain of Gurus whose power exists behind it. OM NAMO (bow, salute) BHAGAVATE (Divine) VASUDEVAY (Lord Krishna). This is a mantra of Bhagavatam (ancient book of Hinduism and Yoga). It was spread by great masters like Vyasa, Shukdev, and Narada. It is mentioned in the Karmakands of Vedas and is called a Vedic Mantra. It is also a mantra of Lord Vishnu (the Sustainer), has twelve letters, and is called Dwadash Akshara Mantra. Prajapati or Creator is Rishi, Vasudeva is Devata, and OM is the Bija Mantra.

OM: It is Nada Brahma, the supreme being, and transcends the barriers of time and language.

NAMO or **NAMAH**: It means bowing of Sashtang Dundavat where six parts of the body touch the floor while bowing. Speech and mind are offered at that time to the supreme being. In the real sense it means surrender of body, mind, heart, and ego to the divine.

BHAGAVATE: This means Godhead and comes from the word Bhagwan or God, Supreme Being. God has six qualities: 1. Aishvarya or mastery and control, 2. Yasha or glory, 3. Veerya or energy, 4. Shree or prosperity, 5. Gnana or knowledge, and 6. Vairagya or non-attachment. These six qualities co-exist in the Godhead, and by repeating this mantra one attracts these qualities to himself.

VASUDEVAY: Vasudev means the Father of the universe. He who lives in all living beings and creatures, and in whom all creatures live homogeneously is called Vasudeva. Through his divine play, Lila, he takes human form to establish order in the world. Lord Krishna is the incarnation of Vasudeva.

MANTRAS USED BEFORE GROUP MEDITATION

OM SAHANA VAVATU SAHANAU BHUNAKTU SAHAVIRYAM KARAVA VAHAI TEJASVINA VADHITAMASTU MA VIDVISHA VAHAI OM SHANTIH SHANTIH SHANTIH

May the eternal guard us all together, may the eternal nourish us all together, may we make bold attempts and adventures together, may our studies and knowledge be illuminative, may we not hate anyone. In the name of the eternal may there be peace, peace, peace. (This mantra may also be used at the end of meditation.)

ASATO MAA SAD GAMAYA TAMASO MAA JYOTIR GAMAYA MRITYOR MAA AMRITAM GAMAYA

Lead me from unreal to real, lead me from darkness to light, lead me from mortality to immortality.

OM POORNAMADAH POORNAMIDAM POORNAT POORNAM UDACHYATE POORNASYA POORNAMADAYA

POORNAMEVA AVASHISHYATE OM SHANTIH SHANTIH
SHANTIH
        That is perfect (whole or full), this is perfect.
This perfect has been projected from that perfect. When this
perfect is subtracted from that perfect the perfect verily remains
perfect. (This is Shanti Patha or Peace Invocation.)

PRAYERS TO GURU

GURUR BRAHMA GURUR VISHNU GURUR DEVO
MAHESHVARAH GURUR SAKSHAT PARABRAHMA
TASMAI SHRI GURAVE NAMAH
        Guru is Brahma, Guru is Vishnu, Guru is
Mahesh (Shiva). Guru is in reality the supreme absolute
Brahma. To the Guru I prostrate.

OM NAMAH SHIVAY GURAVE SATCHIDANANDA
MOORTAYE NISPRAPANCHAY SHANTAY NIRALAMBAY
TEJASE
        Prostration to the Guru who is Shiva, who is the
embodiment of Sat (existence), Chit (knowledge), and Ananda
(bliss), who is free from worldly involvements, peaceful, self-
sustained, and self-effulgent.

MANTRAS FOR SURRENDER

TVAMEVA MATA CHA PITA TVAMEVA TVAMEVA
BANDHU SCHA SAKHA TVAMEVA TVAMEVA VIDYA
DRAVINAM TVAMEVA TVAMEVA SARVAM MAMA DEVA
DEVA
        Thou are my mother and my father. Thou art my
brother and my friend. Thou art my knowledge and my wealth.
Oh Lord of Lords, Thou art my everything.

KAYEN VACHA MANASE NDRIYE VA BUDDHYATMANA
VA PRAKRITES SVABHAVAT KAROMI YADYAD
SAKALAM PARASMAI NARAYANAYETI SAMARPAYAMI
        All that I do by the body, speech, mind, senses,
intellect, soul, or inborn natural tendencies I offer (surrender) to
the supreme Lord Narayana.

ANNAM VAI BRAHMAN DHEEMAHI PRANAM VAI
BRAHMAN DHEEMAHI MANASAM VAI BRAHMAN

DHEEMAHI VIGNANAM VAI BRAHMAN DHEEMAHI
ANANDAM VAI BRAHMAN DHEEMAHI
This food sheath (gross body) is Brahman
(Supreme Being). This vital sheath (prana in the body) is
Brahman. The mental sheath is Brahman. The intellect sheath is
Brahman and the bliss sheath is verily Brahman. (It is used for
affirmation of "I am Brahman" and to remove the wrong
identification of the Self as the body, mind, or ego. Also,
surrender each sheath while meditating.)

MANTRAS USED BEFORE EATING

OM TAT SAT BRAHMARPANA MASTU
OM, That is reality. Let everything be offered to
God. (This mantra is chanted orally or mentally before
commencing any activity like eating, reading, working, etc. One
offers the Divine the actions and results and becomes free from
the karmas.)

BRAHMARPANAM BRAHMA HAVIR BRAHMAGNAU
BRAHMANA HOOTAM BRAHMAIV TENA GANTAVYAM
BRAHMA KARMA SAMADHINA
Brahman is the instrument of oblation, the fire,
the material of oblation (ghee) and the act of oblation. The one
who sees Brahman in all activities attains Brahman.

VEDIC OR MOKSHA MANTRAS
(Mantras for Liberation)

OM
SO HUM (I am That.)
HARI OM
SHIVO HUM (I am Shiva)
AHUM BRAHMASMI (I am Brahman)
OM TAT SAT (That is reality)
OM TAT TWAM ASI (Thou art that)

All of the above Vedic Mantras help to remove the
wrong identification about the Self. They are chanted mentally
while meditating on their meaning. They are also called liberation
or positive affirmation mantras.

GAYATRI MANTRA

OM BHOOR BHUVAH SWAHA TAT SAVITUR VARENYAM
BHARGO DEVASYA DHEEMAHI DHIYO YO NAH
PRACHODAYAT.

We meditate on God's glory, who has created the universe, who deserves worshiping, who is the embodiment of knowledge and light, who is the remover of all sins and ignorance. May He enlighten our intellects.

Gayatri is the mother of the Vedas, Vishvamitra is the rishi, Savita is the presiding deity, Gayatri is the metre. The real meaning of Gayatri is the affirmation that *I am the divine being, created in the image of Him.* This mantra fulfills many desires, and the glory of this mantra is described in the Upanishads.

MANTRA FOR ENDING GROUP MEDITATION

SARVETRA SUKHINAH SANTU SARVE SANTU
NIRAMAYA SARVE BHADRANI PASHYANTU MA
KASHCHIT DUKHAM AAPNUYAT

May everyone become happy, may everyone remain healthy, may everyone find peace and good fortune; may none suffer or become unhappy.

MAHA OR UNIVERSAL MANTRAS

Maha means great. These mantras are those with vibrations. They have no intellectual meaning, but contain the holy names of God. The vibrations produced by them are very important. These names are universal names for God. They can be chanted by anyone at any time, alone or in group meditation with clapping and instruments.

HARE KRISHNA HARE KRISHNA, KRISHNA KRISHNA
HARE HARE, HARE RAMA HARE RAMA, RAMA RAMA
HARE HARE

SHIVA HARA SHIVA HARA SHIVA HARA SHIVA HARA,
SAMBA SADA SHIVA HARA HARA HARA HARA

SHRI KRISHNA GOVINDA HARE MURARE HE NATHA
NARAYANA VASUDEVA

RAMA RAGHAVA RAMA RAGHAVA, RAMA RAGHAVA
RAKSHA MAAM KRISHNA KESHAVA KRISHNA
KESHAVA, KRISHNHA KESHAVA PAAHIMAAM

HARI HARI BOL HARI HARI BOL MUKUNDA MADHAV
GOVINDA BOL

MISCELLANEOUS MANTRAS

(Refer to Healing Mantra Chants Volumes 1 and 2 for musical
rendering of most of the mantras in this chapter.)

1. OM NAMAH SHIVAY
2. GOVINDA JAI JAI, GOPALA JAI JAI, RADHA
RAMANA HARI, GOVINDA JAI JAI
3. HARI HARI RADHA KRISHNA GOVINDA
GOPALA VASUDEVA
4. HARI HARI HARI HARI HARI HARI BOL,
MUKUNDA MADHAV GOVINDA BOL
5. NARAYANA NARAYANA OM
6. ANANDO HUM ANANDO HUM ANANDAM
PARAMANANDAM
7. SRI RAM JAI RAM JAI JAI RAM
8. JAI GURU DEVA JAI SATYA GURU DEV
9. OM SHANTI OM SHANTI OM SHANTI OM
10. KRISHNA KRISHNA SO HUM YOUR AND I ARE
ONE, RAMA RAMA SO HUM YOU AND I ARE ONE.
11. RADHE GOVINDA BHAJO RADHE GOVINDA
12. RATA MANA RAMA RATA MANA RAMA RAMA
SITA RAM
13. HARE RAMA RAMA RAM, HARE RAMA RAMA

ARTI

Arti is a devotional service. A devotee symbolically offers the five basic elements from which he is made to the Lord. They are earth, water, fire, air, and ether. Afterwards he accepts them as PRASAD (Blessings of God). This helps him in surrendering his life to God. He works selflessly and dedicates the fruits of his actions to the Lord. One also receives light (fire) with his hands and transfers it to his face. Light represents knowledge and consciousness, which remove the darkness of ignorance (the root cause of suffering).

OM JAYA JAGADISHA HARE PRABHU JAYA JAGADISHA HARE
Glory to the Lord of the Universe! Hail Lord! Glory to the Lord of the Universe!

BHAKTA JANANA KE SANKATA (twice) KSHANAMEH DURA KARE OM JAYA JAGADISHA HARE
He removes the troubles of the devotees in a moment. Glory to the Lord!

JO DHYAVE FALA PAAVE DUKHA VINASHAI MANAKA PRABHU DUKHA VINASHAI MANAKA
He gives the desired fruits to the devotees, and removes the sorrows of hearts.

SUKHA SAMPATA GHARA AAVE (twice) KASHTA MITE TANAKA OM JAYA JAGADISHA HARE
He provides happiness and wealth, and removes physical sufferings. Glory to the Lord!

MATA PITA TUMA MERE SHARANA GRAHUM KISAKI HARI SHARANA GRAHUN KISAKI
Thou art my mother and my father, from whom else can I seek refuge?

TUMA BINA AURA NA DOOJA (twice) AASHA KARUN KISAKI OM JAYA JAGADISHA HARE
There is none except you. In whom else can I hope? Glory to the Lord!

TUMA PURANA PARAMATMA TUMA ANTARYAMI
PRABHU TUMA ANTARYAMI
Thou art perfect Parmatma. Thou art the knower of all hearts.

PAARA BRAHMA PARAMESHVARA (twice) TUMA
SABAKE SWAMI OM JAYA JAGADISHA HARE
Thou art beyond Brahma. Supreme Lord. Thou art the master of
all. Glory to the Lord!

TUMA KARUNA KE SAAGAR TUMA PAALANA KARTA
PRABHU TUMA PAALANA KARTA
Thou art the ocean of mercy. Thou art the protector of all.

MAI MOORAKHA KHALA KAMI (twice) KRIPA KARO
BHARATA OM JAYA JAGADISHA HARE
I am the ignorant and passionate. Have mercy on me. Glory to
the Lord!

TUMAHI EKA AGOCHARA SABAKE PRANAPATI
PRABHU SABAKE PRANA PATI
Thou art unseekable and protector of all life.

KISA BIDHA MILUN DAYAMAYA (twice) TUMAKO MAI
KUMATI OM JAYA JAGADISHA HARE
Merciful one, I am full of ignorance. How can I find you?
Glory to the Lord!

DEENA BANDHU DUKHA HARTA TUMA RAKSHAKA
MERE SWAMI TUMA RAKSHAKA MERE
Brother of the meek, reliever of sorrow, thou art my protector.

KARUNA HASTA BADHAO (twice) SHARANA PADA TERE
OM JAYA JAGADISHA HARE
Extend your merciful hand. I am at your feet. Glory to the Lord!

VISHAYA VIKARA MITAO PAPA HARO DEVA MERE
PAPA HARO DEVA
Remove my passions and temptations. Oh God, remove my
ignorance.

SHRADDHA BHAKTI BADHAO (twice) SANTANA KI SEVA
OM JAYA JAGADISHA HARE

Increase my devotion, faith, and service to the saints. Glory to the Lord!

Leader: BOLO SHREE SADGURU   Group: DEVA KI JAI
Leader: BOLO SHREE SHREEKRISHNA CHANDRA
Group: BHAGAWAN KI JAI
Together: OM NAMO PARVATI PATE HARA HARA MAHADEV
Glory to the Guru, Glory to the Lord. Glory, glory to the Supreme Lord !!!!!!!

Eyes are the mirrors of the soul. Learn to look into the eyes of a person and learn to feel his vibrations. Learn to communicate in silence instead of superficial words.

Most people get excited from external stimulation. When the stimulation stops they become bored. Use this boredom as an opportunity for inner exploration and to find inner joy.

Be committed to the goal and not to the means. Be committed to experience and not to belief. Be committed to love but do not be attached to loved ones.

Roasted seeds do not sprout. Activities (karmas) produced without attachments and ego do not bind you.

We have limited time in a day. If you want to accomplish something, set priorities.

12

SURRENDER YOGA

Sharanagati Yoga is the Yoga of Surrender to the divine. It gives the aspirant direct communion with divine powers which guide and protect him. Surrender usually implies defeat; giving up because of weakness. Here, however, surrender means that one opens up, merges and expands. The devotee surrenders his body, mind, heart, and ego to the divine Supreme Being and realizes awareness of his true nature, which is the omnipresent and omnipotent Self. This surrender is opening and expanding.

Through surrender the lower nature is transformed into its innate divine nature. As a drop of water merges with the ocean and becomes the ocean, so the aspirant loses identification as an individual being and feels he is part of the whole. This change is a sign of growth. A seed grows into a plant when it submits itself to nature, losing its identification as a seed. By surrender one becomes united with the supreme.

Man has created many luxuries for making his life more comfortable, but these luxuries have also complicated his life. We have fallen out of step with the rhythm of nature, producing a great deal of anxiety. With surrender the internal individual rhythm is re-established with the universal rhythm. The ignorant man carries his luggage on his head while traveling on a train, forgetting that the train is carrying him as well as all of his possessions. The supreme to whom one surrenders is like the train; all burdens are carried by Him and the traveler may relax.

With surrender the seeker realizes that he is only an instrument, not the doer but just a witness. He must play his role in the world like an actor in a play. He performs his duties with love and interest, and surrenders the results of his actions to the Supreme.

Surrendering is opening. One must dive deep within himself, like ocean divers, to find valuable pearls. By traveling in the circles of known concepts growth does not occur. In surrender we must give up all concepts, hopes, fears, expectations, and imaginations in order to grow to our highest potential.

The struggle for perfection may produce tension. There were two yogis meditating. The first yogi was expecting liberation. When he was told that he had only a few years to go before this happened, he was disturbed and was not liberated. The second yogi was content in his practice. When he was told that he had several more lifetimes before liberation, he was still content to be on the path. Because of this attitude he attained quick liberation in the same lifetime. He had surrendered completely. A contented person is liberated quickly. Surrender quickens one's progress.

Most people try to meditate by forcing the body and mind, producing fatigue and tension, and they eventually become disinterested. In surrender meditation one does not force his body or mind, but instead practices the witness technique. When a boat is anchored to the dock, it cannot be paddled to the ocean. In the same way, as long as attention is drawn to pains and awareness of the body and senses, we cannot travel into the deep regions of meditation.

Our body is a physical instrument. Mind is the king and prana (life force) is the minister. Mind directs prana to perform all physical and mental activities. Involuntary activities are independently controlled by prana. Prana would like to lead man to evolution but the mind interferes. In surrender meditation, the control of mind is lifted from the natural flow of prana. This allows prana to take care of the welfare of the body, directing it into suitable positions as needed, while the mind witnesses the whole scene without interference. Prana may cause one to do different postures, mudras, concentration, dancing and singing activities, or it may bring subtle internal changes. The process is very interesting and one looks forward to his regular practice.

As rivers naturally flow towards the ocean, prana naturally rushes from the base of the spine to the thousand petal lotus at the top of the head. The rising of prana (Kundalini awakening) is a sign of evolution. Prana must travel through the middle tube in the spine, piercing the seven chakras (spiritual centers). (See Chapter 8 for details.) The surrender meditation technique purifies the nerves in the body by various postures, mudras, and breathing movements. This prepares one for this Kundalini awakening.

MEDITATION TECHNIQUE

Sit in a comfortable position, keeping the body straight but relaxed. Silently pray to God or Guru for a few moments. Let the mind be free from preoccupation with the past or future. Observe silence and engage the mind in pious thoughts. Your meditation will bring success to the extent of your mental devotion. You will receive Guru's help by being open and receptive.

After that, take twenty slow deep breaths. Then loosen the body by withdrawing control of the mind. The body should not be stiff or tight, as this will prevent the free flow of prana. (Regular Hatha Yoga practice will help maintain a flexible and relaxed body.) When the connection of mind to body is broken, movements are automatically generated in the body, usually within five to ten minutes at the most. Keep the mind occupied with observing the flow of prana in the body, remaining a witness to the inner experience.

Do not stop the movements generated automatically during meditation. The body may begin to bend, or hands and legs may begin to move; just remain a witness and allow the body freedom of movement. Pranayama (breathing technique), weeping, singing, or dancing may begin. Allow the senses and the body complete freedom. As you go deeper into meditation, you will feel separated from your body and will realize that, in spite of the body being active, you are not consciously performing these actions. They are being performed automatically and you are merely a witness.

Ignore background sounds and noises going on around you. Keep your mind engaged in the experiences you are undergoing in meditation. Your eyes should remain closed throughout the process so your concentration is not disturbed. Come out of the meditation slowly, experiencing the after effects and maintaining silence as long as possible.

Several additional suggestions which will help maintain and support your practice: 1. Read inspirational scriptures daily. 2. Observe all Yamas and Niyamas. 3. Try to maintain a regular practice time, morning and/or evening, keeping a brief diary of experiences and mental states during meditation. 4. Do not discuss your experiences with anyone except your Guru or other seekers at your level.

Samadhi is not achieved in a few days or months. One must undergo penance for many years in order to attain samadhi. In Surrender Meditation prana promotes Yoga positions, mudras, yogic breathing, automatic mantra chanting, etc., for many years until all of the astral nerves are purified. Then one goes through mental purification in the form of TANDRA (yogic slumber), YOGA NIDRA (yogic sleep), and MOORCHA (yogic swoon). As one goes through these stages, breathing becomes very slow and the body remains stiff. After passing through these stages, one finally enters Samadhi.

Don't expect to be a Saint overnight. It is easier to feel emotional highs from time to time but harder to maintain a steady feeling for a prolonged time. It is better to integrate smaller disciplines in life, one at a time and with patience, than to expect all the changes to take place on your birthday or New Year's Day.

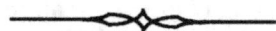

There are many paths to climb a mountain - a long but safe path or a short steep climb. It is hard to climb a mountain but easy to fall. It is hard to be established in disciplines but easy to slide. When you are established in disciplines, keep them up. It is easy to roll with a moving car but harder to push a car which is parked.

Non-attachment is to live fully in the world without being disturbed by it. Be like a lotus leaf which lives in the water but is not touched by it. Live like a tortoise who uses his limbs for prey but withdraws them in time of danger. Non-attachment comes from understanding the transitory nature of the universe all around us. When we understand impermanence, we let go of attachments.

13

GURU

The goal of Yoga is to know thyself. The individual self is the same as the Universal Self or Nirguna Brahman (Impersonal Universal God). To reach this high ideal, the seeker worships a personal God (Idol). A Personal God is an Avatara (Incarnation of Godhead in human form). His idol is worshiped in symbolic form as a picture or statue. However, an even closer association is needed for growth. One needs a medium, and this cannot be provided by symbols or books. Only a soul can inspire and guide another soul. The soul who is on a higher scale of evolution can inspire, guide, and transfer energy to another on a lower scale. This spiritual guide, or teacher, is called a Guru. (Gu-darkness, Ru-light) The Guru leads his disciples from darkness to light.

A lighted candle can light other candles. In the same way, an enlightened Guru can enlighten many souls. The position of a Guru is like the relationship in Christianity of Father, Son, and Holy Ghost. The Holy Ghost makes the contact between Father and Son. In the same way, the Guru makes contact between a shishya (disciple) and his personal deity. As one evolves, the Guru disappears, leaving only the deity and the disciple. Later on the sadhaka (disciple) and the deity become one and inseparable. In the highest evolution, one dissolves the image of the deity into an impersonal, omnipresent God. It is said that when a disciple is ready, the Guru appears. This does not mean that a miracle takes place. Rather it means that one's eyes open and he sees his Guru in persons and situations which could not be seen before.

The Guru is a spiritual teacher and has experienced the higher reality. Having tread the path, he is able to guide his disciple, teaching the truth by the example of his own life. He has no desire to gather many disciples for the purpose of teaching his dogma. Rather, the Guru is an open person, offering his wisdom freely to those who naturally come to him. He does not simply intellectualize but teaches practiccal lessons with compassion to both saints and sinners. The truth is told, though it may be bitter, but it becomes palatable because of his love and compassion for all. For him there is no distinction between saint or sinner, rich or poor. Serving his disciples is like serving God.

Although a Guru is an enlightened person, he is still in the human body and bound by human limitations. A perfectly enlightened Guru is almost impossible to find. Gurus are both practitioners and teachers of Yoga and spend part of their time helping disciples to grow.

There are no set external qualifications for a Guru, therefore one cannot judge and evaluate a Guru. It is individual personal experience that determines the quality of a Guru. He is not determined by the number of followers he has, nor by his fame, but rather by one's individual connection and communication with him. An aspirant should be able to relate individually to his Guru and derive inspiration.

It is a difficult task to become a chela (disciple). People may go shopping for the right Guru and never find him. The seeker must be qualified to find a Guru. An unqualified person may meet an enlightened Guru, yet will not recognize him. For example, a scholar went to a famous Guru to seek knowledge. The Guru served him tea. He poured the tea until the cup began to overflow, and then explained to the shocked scholar that he must empty his mind of all intellectual concepts in order to receive knowledge and wisdom.

The first requirement in becoming a disciple is open-mindedness. The mind is like a container. A gallon jug cannot hold any more water than a gallon even if one immersed it in a lake or ocean. Likewise, knowledge from a Guru is received according to the disciple's amount of openness. The second qualification is to develop patience. A person without patience will be changing paths, goals, and Gurus like a man searching for water, digging many shallow holes and not finding water. Find the proper spot for digging a well by studying the land and seeking expert advice. Once the spot is determined, one should keep digging until water is found. Similarly, one should choose a proper Guru by looking at his purity and character. His presence should be soothing and inspirational.

After finding a Guru, leave your life in his hands. Serve him constantly, obey and respect him as a living God. The Guru is like Brahma, Vishnu, and Mahesh combined. His teachings do not come by formal lectures but by his blessings. The most vital teachings of a Guru come in a very casual manner and an alert disciple catches these teachings immediately. The

Guru transfers his spiritual energy to his disciple knowingly or unknowingly while he is served by the disciple with humility. Although the Guru is in human form, performing human activities, at certain times he is capable of attunement to higher sources of energy and becomes a channel for transferring this energy to his disciples. An evolved and pure Guru will never make any claim to such powers. He can transfer his energy by touch, sight, and even by thought. Many times a disciple may receive energy from his Guru merely by staying in his physical presence.

The disciple should keep his Guru's image on his altar and in his heart as this will provide him with constant guidance, inspiration, and love. A Guru is a psychic person and knows his disciple inside out. He knows what is best for him better than the disciple himself. Do not doubt the Guru's word or his character even if it does not look rational at the time. Be completely open to your Guru and discuss all intimate problems with him without reservation. Many disciples feel guilty and run from their Guru due to this feeling of guilt and weakness. This hinders the disciple's progress, but the Guru is always merciful and forgiving and will give strength to his disciple.

A pure Guru does not try to control his disciple, nor does he try to make him dependent. Rather, he gives him strength to stand on his own feet. The Guru is like a railway engine, the disciple is like a train car. Coupled to his Guru, a disciple is guided by his energy.

In ancient times, disciples spent Brahmacharyashrama (first twenty-five years of life) with the Guru, serving him and his family while studying under him. This relationship was unconditional. The Guru initiated the disciple at the end of his education with the proper mantra, according to the disciple's psychological tendencies. Before one tries unconditional love in the world, he should experience unconditional love with his Guru. Egotistical people and those with narrow minds do not believe in having a Guru. Very highly evolved souls may do without a specific Guru. Saint Dattatreya found birds, bees, flowers, and ants to be his Gurus. The average person, however, needs a Guru for quickening his spiritual growth.

14

INITIATION (DIKSHA)

Initiation (Diksha) is the holiest and most significant of the sacred rituals in the spiritual life of an aspirant. Diksha is a spiritual rebirth for an aspirant where his life style and values change, and he starts living a richer, fuller, and more harmonious life. Another word for Diksha is Abhisheka which means pouring and signifies the pouring of a Guru's energy into his Chela (initiate). Initiation establishes the spiritual communion between Guru and Chela. A Chela should prepare himself as a vessel to receive the Guru's energy, which is constantly flowing. He prepares himself to receive this energy by opening up prior to initiation.

The Guru is similar to the sun which shines and rain that falls indiscriminately. The disciple can be compared to a field which needs to be ploughed and then properly seeded in order to take advantage of the sun and rain. If one is not prepared, the seeds will be washed away with the rain.

Initiation is given by an evolved Guru who has tread the spiritual path and can guide his Shishya. He is like a railway engine and the Shishya is like a railway car. Through initiation the Shishya links himself to his Guru with the chains of faith, love, and devotion. He is constantly guided by his Guru like a cart that is pulled by an engine.

In the earlier stages of the spiritual path, the seeker is curious and is searching for direction. He may change paths and become confused. When a proper Guru is found and the aspirant is completely settled in his goals, he should take initiation from his Guru. The Guru will guide him into a narrow, specific path in order to channelize the disciple's energy. After initiation, one should focus on his path, yet retain full acceptance of those who follow different paths. One should stick to his path with patience and non-attachment to progress.

Real initiation comes when one is opened up completely. Because the changes are internal and subtle, do not expect to be changed overnight by taking initiation. With initiation one takes a new, fresh direction. It is not joining a club to avoid loneliness, or to inflate one's ego by belonging to a specific group. Such external changes as receiving a new name or changing the style of clothing are symbolic and serve only to remind one of his spiritual rebirth.

Some people may use initiation as an escape from responsibilities, or may become too dependent on the Guru. If one seeks and accepts initiation prematurely, he may feel guilty for his commitment if he does not pursue his practice. This guilt may make him abandon his practice completely. An initiate should stay in constant touch with his Guru for his assistance and guidance on the path.

At the time of initiation the Guru gives a specific mantra to the initiate. This mantra is called the Guru Mantra and should be repeated constantly whenever possible. The Guru Mantra generates the Guru's strength and should be used for spiritual guidance when the Guru is not available.

OM NAMO BHAGAVATE VASUDEVAY

We should not look at the finger of a master, but we should look at where it is pointing.

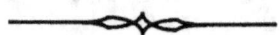

Human life is precious. One-third of life is spent in sleeping, youth is spent in playing, middle years go by in worldly pursuits, old age brings sickness and suffering. Unless we wake up and choose to find Self-realization, life will quickly pass us by.

We are hiding under masks of our desires, attachments, wishes, fears, and prejudices. We can be free as soon as we take off the masks and realize that we are free. There is nothing to do - no place to go - nothing to be.

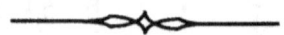

15

GNANA YOGA

The goal of Gnana Yoga is <u>Know Thyself</u>. This is the highest goal and highest knowledge that a human being can attain. After experiencing the Self, the mysteries of life are unfolded and all human goals and ambitions are fulfilled. Other knowledge in the universe can be represented as zeros which have no value of their own until the number one is placed in front of them. Self-knowledge functions as this number one, giving value to everything else.

Gnana means knowledge or wisdom. Gnana Yoga is the path to attain union with the Supreme Lord through knowledge and wisdom. This is a suitable path for persons with logical and intellectual tendencies.

Gnana Yoga uses discrimination techniques. One uses the purified and sharp mind to discriminate between real and unreal, permanent and impermanent. When one understands the permanence of his own Self through direct and personal experience, he rises above all illusions, attains the highest kind of peace, and becomes free. After attaining this wisdom the yogi continues to function in the world with absolute freedom. Desires and karmas no longer bind him; he takes life as a play or mirage and rises above all dualities.

The average person receives knowledge and perceptions objectively. This type of knowledge is relative because it is subject to time, space, and causation. As knowledge is filtered through the mind, it becomes contaminated, twisted, and distorted, depending upon many factors. Gnana Yogi seeks subjective knowledge. There is no mind to interfere as subject, object, and method of perception all merge. The knower, known, and knowledge become one.

THE GNANA YOGA PATH

Gnana Yoga is the straightest and most direct path of Yoga. This path is extremely difficult for the average person to practice. Most people can follow the initial stages of Gnana Yoga, deriving many practical benefits, but the advanced Gnana

Yoga path requires cleansing of body and mind with the practice of other branches of Yoga.

Initial inquiries of Gnana Yoga begin with rational analysis of the conscious mind to find out, "Who am I?" One analyzes his body, senses, thoughts, emotions, and behavior scientifically with an open mind. All preconceived ideas, dogmas, blind faith, rituals, and superstitions are removed, and reliance is placed on personal experience. With the technique of negation, everything is rejected that is not permanent or non-Self. As the wind removes clouds from the sky, revealing the sun, Neti, Neti, (I am not this, I am not that) is a technique which removes the veils of maya and eventually the Self becomes visible. After removing all negatives which are non-Self, the person meditates and tunes into his inner center to experience his real essence: "I am That", or "I am Brahman" (Ahum Brahmasmi).

There are fundamental questions concerned with life: Who am I? Where do I come from? What is my destiny? How was the universe created? Who sustains this universe? These questions were asked in the past and will continue to be asked again and again. This fundamental puzzle exists in everyone's mind. One tries to hide and run from these inquiries by following the path of transitory happiness. Like a caterpillar, he produces a network of illusions around him for happiness, but the same illusions eventually trap and destroy him. Death, however, does not leave anyone untouched. Persons of wisdom try to solve this puzzle before their time is up, as they know that human birth is not without meaning. The seers solved the puzzle using their bodies and minds as laboratories, and they spent their entire life searching for the truth. Their experiences are revealed in the Upanishads.

The mystery is not revealed, however, by reading, discussion, or mere intellectual understanding. One must experience the higher reality face to face. Trying to describe this experience is like talking to a blind person about the colors in the sky. Scriptures provide the direction for the search, but one must put into practice the teachings of the scriptures and suggestions of the great saints rather than merely intellectualizing. Hunger cannot be satisfied by looking at or thinking about food, it must be eaten.

SCRIPTURAL AUTHORITY

According to Vedanta, Gnana Yoga utilizes inquiry using the Buddhi (intellect) which is sharper than the edge of a razor. Katha Upanishad explains that one who has not turned away from bad conduct, whose senses are not under control, and whose mind is not at rest, cannot attain Atman (the Self) by means of intelligence. Atman is attainable by the love of truth, by austerity, by correct knowledge, and a life of chastity which is constantly practiced. Scriptures and intellectual inquiries are preliminary preparations for higher inquiry which takes place in samadhi (complete absorption in meditation) and is subjective knowledge.

The ten major Upanishads reveal Gnana Yoga in the form of experiences of the seers. The Bhagavad Gita explains Gnana Yoga in the second chapter. Brahma Sutra, written by Badarayana is a direct inquiry of Brahman. Gnana Yogi Shankara of the 9th century A.D. is the authoritative interpreter of the Brahma Sutras. His own literature, Viveka Chudamani (Crest Jewel of Discrimination) and Upadesha Sahashri are very logical text books of Gnana Yoga for modern man.

OUR WORLD OF ILLUSION

The goal of Gnana Yoga is to "know thyself." Where is this Self? It is closer than the closest, yet we do not know it. It is our very Self and life yet we cannot see it, and we run around like a musk deer in the jungle of desires in search of the fragrance of happiness. Self is the most precious thing that we have, yet we pawn that diamond for the shiny stones of worldly happiness. Shankara explains that Brahman (the Universal Self) or Atman (Individual Self) is real and that Jagat (apparent universe that we perceive with our senses) is an illusion. Brahman is Sat (pure existence), Chit (pure knowledge), and Anand (bliss). Brahman is real and does not change or cease to exist. The world exists in time and space, is constantly changing, is subject to cause and effect, but Brahman remains as the unchanging essence of everything.

In normal conditions we experience three states of consciousness: waking, dreaming, and dreamless sleep. Our experiences in these three different states contradict one another. In samadhi one experiences higher consciousness called Turiya, a fourth state. This is the total consciousness which transcends the three lower states. In the Turiya state one experiences the Self (Atman) to uniquely exist beyond time, space, and causation. In darkness one sees a snake in a rope and becomes frightened, but when the light is turned on, the snake disappears. In the same way, under the dark spell of maya (cosmic illusion) one identifies himself with the limited self. As soon as the experience of the real Self is attained, ignorance disappears. The dream seems real to the dreamer so he suffers the consequences of his experience, but as soon as he wakes up, he ignores the dream knowing it to be an illusion.

The world we live in is also a cosmic dream. You are dreaming right now and accepting everything as real. The world, of course, is relatively real in the lower states of consciousness. When we wake up into the higher consciousness of samadhi, however, we realize that this world is also a dream. All our possessions, ambitions, and attachments, which we consider very real, are similar to a child playing with his toys believing them to be real. An adult loses his attachment for toys as he develops attachment to more important things in life. In the same way, attachment to material life falls off after experiencing the Self. Maya is a cosmic illusion. The power of maya veils the experience of Brahman so that infinite Brahman seems to be the finite world of our existence. This finite world is superimposed upon Brahman like the rope that appeared to be a snake in the darkness.

THE NATURE OF MAYA

Maya is cosmic illusion. It covers Brahman like clouds cover the sun. It is without beginning and was created by ignorance. Ignorance and maya are causes of each other, like the chicken and the egg, or a seed and the tree. We cannot determine which came first. The only explanation we can envision is to consider it to be Lila (a Divine play).

The concept of maya is similar to the concept of Prakriti of Samkhya Yoga. (See chart in Chapter 2.) It has three qualities: 1. Satva (purity), 2. Rajas (activity), and 3. Tamas (inertia). We exist in maya. At the individual level maya is called AVIDYA (ignorance). Avidya has no beginning but there is the possibility to rise above it. When we purify ourselves and function at <u>Satva</u> level we can transcend maya and attain Self-knowledge.

When Rajas (activity) is predominant, maya uses the power of projection to generate the phenomenal universe having various names, forms, and limitations. For example, gold is seen as different ornaments instead of gold, and living beings are seen as male, female, animals, or humans, rather than as sparks of God containing the essence of Brahman. This illusion power produces suffering.

When Tamas (inertia) is predominant, maya uses veiling power. This power hides the true essence of the Self. Perceived objects are identified as Perceiver (Self). For example, one identifies himself with his body, mind or emotions. One becomes attached to the world and forgets the true nature of Self, thereby producing suffering.

Brahman and maya have three common characteristics: 1. existence, 2. cognizance, and 3. attractiveness. Brahman is free from names, forms, cause and effect, while maya has these attributes. The finite world of maya functions according to the law of Karma (cause and effect) while Brahman is free. Ego is the cause of the finite universe which separates one's Self from the universe. Ego starts the subject-object relationship. When ego disappears the apparent world also disappears. Ego identifies itself with the body and mind. This identification is created because: 1. It is the nature of ego, 2. Due to past karma, and 3. Due to ignorance. Because of wrong identification a person gets caught up in the veils of maya and forgets his true nature. The pure Self (Atman), contaminated by ego, mind, and desires, becomes jiva (soul). This soul tries to fulfill desires by choosing a suitable body.

All impressions (samskaras) are retained by the mind which provides the soul with the propelling force to continue the journey from life to life in accordance with the law of karma and reincarnation. (See Chapter 16.) Maya offers a choice of two paths: sreya (good) and preya (pleasant). The ignorant choose the path of preya which gives temporary enjoyment but creates the bondage of karma, birth and death, and produces suffering on a longer range. Because of maya, one builds castles in the sand which the waves of time wash away. A person plans his life but has no control over any moment in the future. The wise person, however, chooses the path of sreya (good) and searches for liberation by giving up worldly enjoyment. He attains Self-realization and freedom.

Gnana Yoga

ISHVARA

Brahman is the absolute (universal) aspect of God that encompasses everyone and everything. Since our total being is part of Brahman, our limited mind cannot perceive Brahman. When the mind is dissolved and becomes homogeneous with Brahman, one will experience Brahman. Those who have this experience cannot explain it. Those who talk about it do not know Him (Brahman).

Brahman is the cause and maya is the effect. Being under the influence of maya, we can only see a part of Brahman. It is similar to looking at the ocean and seeing only to the horizon. In devotion we personify Brahman (Impersonal God) and make Him Ishvara (Personal God). The concept of Ishvara is similar to the concept of Purusha in Samkhaya philosophy. (Refer to the chart in Chapter 2.) This personified Brahman is called Ishvara who is the ruler of maya, whereas the individual soul (jiva) is the servant of maya. Ishvara is the highest concept of perfection that the human mind can perceive and that the human heart can love. All religions have Ishvara, a Godhead (Avatara), whom they worship and whom they consider the almighty creator of the universe. In Bhakti Yoga we worship a personal God, Ishvara. In Gnana Yoga one rises above Ishvara and experiences Brahman, the impersonal aspect of God.

****

Two kinds of power exist in maya: vidya or right knowledge, which takes one towards the Self (Brahman), and avidya or ignorance, which takes one away from the Self. Vidya and avidya work together to produce the sum total of good and evil karma. We experience the effect from our karma while producing new karma according to our desires, ultimately reaching Brahman when all illusions dissolve.

Most people do not know their higher nature (true Self). They are caught up in their physical self which is a small reflection of the real Self. Our body is like a lamp. The nerves are the wires, prana is the electricity, mind is the switch, and the Self is the powerhouse which provides energy to all lower manifestations. The Self (Brahman or Atman) shines like a sun providing energy to our causal body, then to our astral body, and finally to our gross body. Atman and Brahman are identical. There is only one sun, yet it reflects in many pools of water and appears to be many suns. In the same way, each individual soul (jiva) reflects Brahman and is called Atman.

MANIFESTATIONS

Our lowest manifestation is in the form of gross body, then astral body, and then causal body. Beyond them all exists Brahman or Atman. We function with all three bodies and there is no distinct line among them. The gross body can be compared to an ice cube, the astral body is like water, and the causal body like vapor. Like the ice cube, the gross body is solid and has a definite size, shape, and limitations. The astral body, like water, has greater fluidity, flexibility, and strength. The causal body, like vapor, is the subtlest and most powerful of all.

We use all three bodies according to our awareness and spiritual growth. In the normal waking state we function with the gross body. In moments of thinking and dreaming we use the astral body, while in deep slumber and deep meditation we use the causal body. In samadhi we transcend all bodies and experience our own pure Atman.

BODY SHEATHS

Our bodies are divided into five sheaths (koshas) (See Figure 1, p. 137.) which are produced by maya. As we grow on the higher path, we peel off one layer of ignorance at a time until we reach our center. What do we find then? We find nothing but a vacuum, but this vacuum which is called Shunyam, is everything. Therefore, we are nothing and everything at the same time. It is described in an Upanishad that a master asks his disciple to get a fruit and open it. The disciple finds the seed inside and when he breaks it he finds nothing. The master then explains that the tree comes from the seed and the subtle essence behind the seed is the essence in which all things have their existence. That is the truth and that is the Self. That art Thou.

The five body sheaths are connected by a subtle cord as long as one is alive in the human form. At the time of death the gross body is cut off from the others. The astral and causal bodies survive after death and subsequently obtain another gross body according to one's own karma.

Gross Body The gross body is made of the food sheath (annamaya kosha) and the vital air sheath (pranamaya kosha). The physical body is the food sheath as it comes into existence and is sustained by food, returning to food (earth) at the time of death. Its characteristics are: birth, death, disease, and decay. Its stages are youth, maturity, and old age. It is made of bone, marrow, fat, blood, skin, etc. and in the subtle sense it contains five basic elements which are earth, water, fire, air, and ether. It contains five organs of action and five organs of perception. The organs of action are hands, legs, speech, excretion, and reproduction. The organs of perception are eyes, nose, ears, tongue, and skin.

Vital air sheath: The air we breathe mixes with the blood and reaches every cell in the physical body. This sheath controls the organs of action and the sense organs. The air sheath is comprised of pancha (five) prana, consisting of five different forms of prana: 1. prana, located between the throat and heart, controls the vocal functions, respiration, seeing, and hearing. 2. apana, located between the navel and the base of the spine, controls the autonomic functions of excretion and reproduction. 3. samana, located in the abdominal region, controls digestion and assimilation. 4. udana, which directs the soul's journey at the time of death, is located above the throat and controls the autonomic functions of the areas above the throat. 5. vyana pervades the entire body through 72,000 nerve channels and controls the basic voluntary and involuntary functions of the body. There are five Upa pranas (secondary pranas) which control some minor functions in the body such as sneezing, hiccups, yawning, etc.

Astral Body The astral body is made up of the mental sheath (manomaya kosha) and the intellectual sheath (vignana maya kosha). The mental sheath contains the mind which experiences emotions, desires, happiness, and is subtler than the food sheath. The intellectual sheath forms doubts, and evaluates and judges situations. It is higher and subtler than the mind because it can venture into realms unheard of or unseen. This subtle body is the seat of our desires.

Causal body The causal body is the bliss sheath (ananda maya kosha), which is made of ignorance and negativity. It is the state beyond waking and dreaming. One's concepts of being rich or poor, happy or unhappy, dissolve into a state of non-apprehension. One may attain the lower phase of it in the slumber state or unconsciousness, or attain positive bliss in samadhi through the mastery of Yoga. Figure 1 shows the connection of the body sheaths to the Absolute Self.

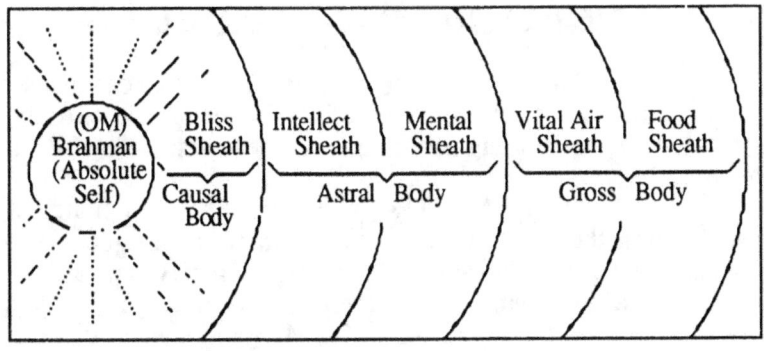

Figure 1

MEDITATION TECHNIQUE NO. 1

Prepare for meditation with the yogic breathing as usual, then chant the following five mantras and absorb the feeling of unity with Brahman.

1. ANNAM VAI BRAHMAN DHIMAHI
This food sheath or gross body is verily Brahman.
2. PRANAM VAI BRAHMAN DHIMAHI
This prana sheath is verily Brahman.
3. MANASAM VAI BRAHMAN DHIMAHI
This mind sheath is verily Brahman.
4. VIGNANAM VAI BRAHMAN DHIMAHI
This intellectual sheath is verily Brahman.
5. ANANDAM VAI BRAHMAN DHIMAHI
This bliss sheath is verily Brahman.

Using this technique, one may let go of himself and of the strong bonds of identification with the body, mind, etc. and may relax enough to do the positive affirmation: AHUM BRAHMASMI (I AM BRAHMAN). It means that I AM sat, pure existence, chit, pure consciousness, and ananda, pure bliss. I am without size or shape, I am free from the bonds of time and space, life and death. I am omnipresent, omnipotent, and omniscient Self. Stay in this ecstasy. This will remove all the veils of maya, and one will experience the Self here and now.

MEDITATION TECHNIQUE NO. 2

This is a more elaborate technique that can be used for problem solving. It may be used in quiet meditation or during the day while performing activities and experiencing the effect of maya.

QUIET MEDITATION: Prepare for meditation as usual, using the breathing and other suitable techniques. Ask yourself mentally: Who am I? Allow time to receive and analyze the answers. Stay with this until you resolve that I am not this. For example: Am I Mr. or Miss X? My name can be changed yet I won't be changed. Am I father, son, brother, or friend? These identifications are only in relation to different situations. I am a father to someone, while a brother to someone else. Am I this gross body with arms, legs, and different organs? I will remain the same even if I lose parts of my body. Can I define myself with the size, weight, and description of my physical structure? The body gains and loses weight and goes on aging. Cells are continually changing their structure, still the awareness of I remains equally strong. I should be beyond the body. Am I these senses? The senses see, hear, smell, taste, and touch, but they see and experience through the mind.

Sometimes a person does not see with wide open eyes when he is absorbed in hearing something or vice versa. In a dream we experience the senses while there is no object of the senses. We may smell or hear and experience pleasure or pain without the presence of the objects of pleasure or pain. Am I the mind? Mind is the cause of time and space, the instrument of perception and learning. It is the cause of emotions, but our beliefs, emotions, and judgments about people and situations change constantly. Our mood changes from hour to hour. We feel happy or unhappy, excited or depressed, yet there is an entity witnessing all the changes of emotions. There is I consciousness which witnesses. This ego must be I, a simple consciousness of existence and awareness which is beyond the mind.

Time and space exist as long as the mind exists. In the physical world time and space are represented by the distance between two events and two objects respectively. Time and space are relative. In the absence of mind the ego is neither male nor female. There is no concept of you and I, and no more separateness. There is only one existence. The concept of you and I is an illusion. Problems are created by holding onto the body and mind which are not real. We must learn to lose ourselves in meditation, service, or devotion. We must lose our limited self to gain the real Self. Stay attuned to your real Self and experience everything as a witness. Experience healing at all levels.

Now sit silently and analyze your everyday situations, your goals, and the activities which make you happy or unhappy. See the transitory nature of all the things of the world. Realize emotions to be petty in comparison to the vast existence of pure consciousness. Know that pleasure and pain are constantly revolving in a circle like a wheel, then witness and transcend them, being at the center. You will eventually grow out of the grip of maya. The center is free from motion but the points on the circumference travel constantly. Similarly, the person who has found the center is free from the grip of birth and death, while others continue to revolve from life to life until they find freedom.

ACTIVE MEDITATION: During the day be aware of your breathing and be a witness to all situations without judging or analyzing. For example, witness the tired body. Witness that the stomach is hungry, the mouth is talking, and the mind is thinking. This awareness will reduce restlessness, thus conserving energy, and will lift you above compulsive habits. This technique can be applied during the day while working, talking, or walking. Be fully aware of each situation and remain a witness of yourself, your activities, and the reactions you have from people and situations. Awareness itself will serve as a torchlight to reveal and eliminate many problems before they begin. Most problems exist because of one's lack of awareness. Witness honors and insults, pleasures and pains, and see the transitory nature of situations. Expand your vision over a longer period. For example, if you are upset with a problem, how will this problem feel one week, one month, or one year from now? The intensity of the problem disappears when it is projected into the future with right awareness. Apply the analysis in the case of physical pain: I am not this body and I am witnessing this situation. This will help to eliminate the pain.

One can also practice identifying with the situation in order to be free from suffering. Problems and suffering are magnified by resistance to situations. Become one with the suffering, one with heat or cold or fears, and be free. Emotional problems can be solved by proper analysis. Use balance and moderation in every activity. Like a tortoise who uses his limbs for catching his prey but withdraws them in times of danger, we should use the same wisdom. A fish is caught due to attraction to taste; a moth is destroyed due to attraction to light; a bee is destroyed due to the attraction to smell; a cobra is caught due to the attraction to music, and an elephant is caught due to the attraction to touch. Utilize awareness and wisdom so you are not caught in the trap of the senses.

The Bhagavad Gita describes Gnana Yoga in the second chapter. It explains the real character of the Atman which is neither created nor destroyed; it is eternal and everlasting and survives when the body dies. The Atman changes the body like changing a garment. We should not grieve for the living nor for the dead because death is like a longer dream. Death of the gross body is inevitable.

The Atman is not wet by water, burned by fire, nor slain by the sword. All work is performed by the three Gunas of Prakriti (nature). We are only the witness, but by identifying with the Gunas we become the doer and, therefore, responsible for all actions. This puts us in the cycle of birth and death. Maintain equilibrium like the depths of an ocean which do not become affected by a turbulent or calm surface. In the same way, maintain emotional balance towards the situations of life. This state is called Sthita Pragnya.

Live a normal life but do not allow situations to overpower you. Be like a lotus leaf that lives on the water, yet water does not touch it.

****

COSMOLOGY

The Samkhya system explains cosmology. (See Chapter 2.) Creation has no absolute beginning. Cosmic energy alternates between evolution (creation) and involution (dissolution). Evolution is called the Day of Brahma (the creative energy of God), and involution is called the Night of Brahma. Cosmic energy consists of three gunas. When the equilibrium of the three gunas is disturbed, it generates universal intelligence, universal ego, mind, organs of action and perception, and the five basic elements. When the elements of the cosmic energy combine in various ways, all beings come into existence: plants, insects, animals, humans, demigods, angels, and spirits.

According to Hindu mythology, the God of creation (Brahma) felt a stir in his consciousness. It produced a full lotus from his navel within which were all the materials for the creation of the universe. Brahma had the desire for knowledge and prayed to the supreme Lord. The Lord commanded him to create the universe as he had done in the past. Brahma entered the heart of the lotus and divided it into three sections, namely: heaven, earth, and sky. He brought out the highest knowledge in the form of four Vedas, representing himself by the sacred syllable and Mantra AUM (OM). With his yogic powers he created the first humans who were deeply involved in meditation and showed no possibility of propagation. Therefore, he divided himself into male and female forms and propagated the universe. The first man was Manu from which the word Manushya, or man, is derived. Manu is the father of mankind. The first woman was called Shatrupa.

The cycle of evolution was divided into four Yugas (ages). 1. Satya Yuga was the age of truthfulness and morality, consisting of 432,000 x 4 = 1,728,000 years. There existed Satya (truth), Daya (compassion), Bhakti (devotion and love), and Dana (charity). 2. The next age, Treta Yuga, was made of 432,000 x 3 = 1,296,000 years. In this age truth (Satya) was destroyed. 3. The next age was called Dwapara Yuga which was made of 432,000 x 2 = 864,000 years. In this age compassion (Daya) was also destroyed. During this age Lord Krishna was incarnated. 4. Our present age is called Kali Yuga which is made of 432,000 years. Bhakti (devotion) is destroyed in this age, only Dana remains. Lord Kalki is predicted to be incarnated during this age to come in a half-human and half-horse form to destroy evil and the evil doers and to re-establish righteousness. The best path for liberation in Kali Yuga is mantra chanting.

+ + + + + + + + + + +

Focus on the tip of the nose and observe the breath (coming and going). Slow it down to the point where a feather held in front of the nose does not flicker. You will attain mastery of your mind and emotions.

Gnana Yoga

MACROCOSM AND MICROCOSM

Pure universal consciousness is called Purusha which is free, without beginning or end. When Purusha identifies itself with Prakriti and establishes itself as the doer, it becomes bound by karma and reincarnates. The sun reflects in water, yet it is not affected by the attributes of water. In the same way, Purusha is not affected by the attributes of the body. Man is created in the image of God and each individual reflects the presence of this Purusha. If universal Purusha is macrocosm, individual Purusha is microcosm. The human body is made of the same basic five elements as the universe. All the stars, galaxies, and solar systems exist in the human body. By studying himself, one can study the whole universe. Study of a single salt crystal produces knowledge of all the salt of the world. In the same way, one knows everything by knowing himself in the true sense. That is why all the religions of the world preach Know Thyself. By studying and controlling our mind, we can study and control all the minds of the universe. By uniting our own mind to the cosmic mind, we can establish contact with all the minds of the universe. Like a phone making contact with the switchboard operator, one line can make contact with all other lines.

In the human microcosm, our brain represents Brahman. This is the center of the Sahashrara chakra (thousand petal lotus), and this is the first organ which is formed in the human body. Next, the spinal cord is formed in which the center between the eyebrows is the seat of individual consciousness. The throat center is the seat of ether, the heart center is the seat of air, the navel is the fire center, the pelvic center is the place of water, and the base of the spine is the earth center. We have evolved from cosmic energy to the earth element. The goal of each person is to return back to the supreme consciousness, which is our Father.

Maya is powerful. It deludes us. We consider ourselves immortal. We build sandcastles of ambitions and chase the mirage of happiness.

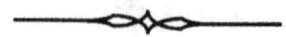

16

REINCARNATION

Yoga traditions hold that Brahman (God, the Absolute) is one without a second and is all pervading. Nothing exists outside of Brahman. Everything is created from it, sustained by it, and dissolves in it. It is without qualities as it is all qualities. This Brahman, or Absolute, is composed of consciousness (Purusha) and matter (Prakriti). The interaction of these forces creates the manifestations of nature which change constantly as interaction changes. Yet, behind all of these changes lies Brahman, the changeless. All we see and experience, therefore, is a manifestation of Brahman. Things change constantly, taking various forms, but the totality remains the same. Nothing new is created and nothing is destroyed. For example, a container of soap solution, depending upon conditions, produces varieties of size and quantities of bubbles, but the soap solution remains constant. The ocean produces varieties of waves but the ocean itself remains unchanged. In the same way, the universe evolves from Brahman and returns to Brahman without affecting Brahman. Energy and souls evolve out of Brahman, manifesting as minerals, plants, micro-organisms, insects, animals, and humans, ultimately returning to Brahman. This process of transmigration is called reincarnation. Only humans have the potential to rise above reincarnation. Yoga provides techniques to reach this goal which is called MOKSHA (liberation). An understanding of reincarnation explains the puzzle of a population explosion. We cannot count the number of humans or animals as they are transforming constantly.

LAW OF PERMANANCE

Modern science supports these yogic principles that nothing can be created or destroyed. For example, wood burns and apparently is destroyed. In reality, however, it has merely been transformed into gaseous products and ashes. Human beings are also subject to this law. Bodies are destroyed and become ashes, but the soul survives and forms another body to fulfill its desires. This is the theory of reincarnation.

In the third chapter of John's Gospel, Christ says: "That which is born of the flesh is flesh, and that which is born of the spirit is spirit. The wind blows where it will and you hear the sound of it. But you do not know whence it comes or whither it goes. So it is for everyone who is born of the spirit."

The soul seems to appear at birth and disappear with death because we cannot see the continuity of its existence. Actually, the soul is like a cable passing through the sea and reappearing at different points. At each point it would appear that there are different cables, but if we trace it from beginning to end, we find one cable, sometimes submerged beneath the ocean, sometimes visible. If we could trace the soul's journey after death we would find the same continuity.

In the Bhagavad Gita Lord Krishna says, "There was never a time when I did not exist, nor you; nor is there any future in which we will cease to be." The soul changes bodies like a person changes garments. When the garment is worn out, we throw it away and take another. The wearer of the garment, however, does not change.

MEMORY OF PREVIOUS LIVES

Various documented proofs of reincarnation are now available. Hypnotists have not only succeeded in regressing subjects to childhood, but have actually regressed them to previous incarnations. Scientific study has proven that children who have recalled events of past lives have been verified with amazing accuracy. This is understandable as children have fewer impressions of their present incarnation to block memories of the past. Some children are born with special gifts or talents which must have been inherited from their previous life. All of us have had feelings about certain places, that we have been there before. We have a certain affinity for some people and feel that we have known them before, because we are easily attracted to them. Also, we feel comfortable with certain philosophies and have inborn convictions that defy all logic. These are indications that we have retained impressions from previous incarnations.

In the state of samadhi yogis have been able to remember their past incarnations. In this state they go beyond time and space to see the continuity of their existence.

Why don't we all remember our past incarnations? God has blessed us by not giving us that faculty. If we could remember our past incarnations indiscriminately we would become confused and mentally disturbed. We only retain the essence of previous incarnations in the form of certain tendencies, convictions, likes, dislikes, ambitions, and desires. This enables us to carry on our present life with enthusiasm and learn the necessary spiritual lessons which we were meant to learn in this particular life.

LAW OF JUSTICE AND ORDER

Probably the greatest support for the idea of reincarnation becomes apparent as we look around. The universe evolves within definite laws; there is no chaos. In nature we find justice and order at all levels and nature is impartial. We have faith in the Lord that he will judge us fairly. Nothing happens by chance or luck, a fact which has been proven by science. We should accept the fact that man is not exempt from this order. All children are born different, some healthy and to prosperous families, others physically handicapped or in poor families. Some children are talented and others are retarded. If there is justice and order in the universe, there must be existence before birth in order to justify the variable conditions at birth. If there is no previous life, then everyone should be born alike and with equal opportunities. The kind of incarnation we take is determined by ourselves. The sum total of all our karmas accumulated through this lifetime, especially our major desires, determines our next incarnation. This process is comparable to choosing suitable clothing for different types of weather. We are able to choose a definite body, environment, and talents which will enable us to fulfill our specific desires.

LAW OF KARMA

If order and justice exist at all, there must be life before birth and after death. This seeming disorder of our visible world is explained by the Law of Karma which goes hand in hand with the concept of reincarnation.

Karma is the law of Ethical Causation. All causes have their effect, and cause and effect are always equal. Thus there is a natural or moral law which maintains an ethical balance at all times. Karma is produced by any activity we perform, whether by thought, speech, or action, with thought being the most powerful of the three. Our life is literally a projection of our own mind. "As ye sow, so shall ye reap." Every activity registers a corresponding impression (samskara) on the mind. More recent impressions remain on the surface, while those of events long past lie buried in the subconscious. We remember what we ate today more clearly than what we ate last week.

There are four kinds of Karmas:

1. SANCHITA KARMA - Accumulated from past incarnations and stored in the subconscious mind.

2. PRARABDHA KARMA - Fate or predestination. It is part of the stored karma that appears in our present life. This explains why some people seem to have good "luck" and others have bad "luck."

3. KRIYAMANA KARMA - Willful actions of the present. We are currently controlling our destiny by choosing our path. We control the steering wheel and brakes of our life and can utilize them as we choose.

4. AGAMI KARMA - Immediate results of our present actions, e.g., if you touch fire you will burn, you experience tension and get a headache, etc.

Cause and effect balance out. If a ball is thrown with a certain force, it will travel the distance in proportion to the energy expended. It travels straight but if a hindrance comes, it changes direction or bounces back. Gravity, air currents, friction, etc. control its destination. The ball stops when energy input and output become equal. In the same way, a physical cause can result in physical, mental, or emotional reactions or a combination of them. A mental or emotional cause can result in a physical, mental, or emotional reaction or a combination. We constantly create new karmas while receiving the results of previous ones. The effect of a first cause can become the cause for the next effect, and a chain reaction continues in a complex manner. These impressions (samskaras) are registered in the subconscious mind.

There are karmas at individual and group levels. Nations and societies have their own group karma. For example, in the United States we are reaping the fruits of our forefather's efforts, and our present actions will determine our children's future. Each new president inherits karma from the previous president.

These karmas function at the universal level and include all other laws of nature and do not contradict them. The laws of physics, metaphysics, genetics, etc. all operate within the Law of Karma. For example, a person inherits his parents' genes, not by chance but by choice as we choose our own parents. This is evidnece that the Law of Karma supercedes all other laws.

The Law of Karma cannot be comprehended completely by our limited mind. We can, however, understand the cause-effect relationship in our life to a great extent, and can extrapolate it to understanding it at the universal level.

Priority of impressions is also important. Some strong or shocking event from childhood may be recalled more clearly than a less important event of the recent past. These impressions are in the mind, dictating much of our present action, and consequently many of the circumstances we encounter in life. Thus persons who enjoy good fortune despite bad deeds are benefitting from previous good karma, while accumulating bad karma (or mental impressions causing personality and habit patterns) for the future. This explains why some good and spiritual people suffer many hardships while some immoral and evil people enjoy good fortune in life.

Karmic debts must always be paid. We can pay them like a mortgage, either in large installments over a short period of time, or in small installments over a longer period of time. There is always perfect justice in the universe and we must eventually pay our debts. We can escape from man-made laws but no one can escape the punishment or reward of his own conscience. These so-called debts may take the form of physical surroundings, dreams, disease (physical or psychological) and guilt complexes. Because the mind is a totally accurate computer for registering karma, we are always sure to get exactly what we deserve.

At the time of death the sum total of good and bad karma remains with the soul and determines the circumstances of his next life and of his existence between physical births. If one has not learned the necessary lessons of a particular lifetime he must repeat his experiences until he evolves higher. It is similar to a child who has not learned the lessons of the 4th grade and must repeat that year until he is ready for 5th grade.

LIFE AFTER DEATH

At the time of death the essence of our entire life's real desires comes to the surface. The last moment of death determines the journey of the soul. We cannot, however, expect to remember God at the moment of death if we have not remembered Him most of our life. Our whole life is a preparation for our journey in the next lifetime. Yogis who have mastery of their life leave their body willfully through the ninth gate (the thousand petal lotus in the skull) and attain liberation.

Some souls become trapped in lower worldly desires and attachments and become ghosts. Ghosts are souls without a body, existing in the earth region. Some souls who have done good deeds go to the higher astral regions and enjoy the pleasures of heaven. Those souls who have done bad deeds go to the lower astral regions and suffer the pains of hell. Most people have mixed karmas and therefore they experience both heaven and hell.

Heavens are enjoyed as long as good karmas last, and hell continues as long as bad karmas last. Ultimately one must return to earth for learning spiritual lessons. Only in human form do we have the potential for enlightenment. For this reason, human birth is considered to be very precious. Souls who have an intense desire to attain a certain mission may take another appropriate body immediately. Others stay in the astral plane for a longer period of rest and learning until they choose to reincarnate.

Can we regress to animal life? It is very unlikely. We always evolve and graduate to higher grades. We could, however, temporarily regress to lower forms of life to learn some lessons, to fulfill some animal desires, or because of our attachments.

The experience in the astral plane is similar to the experience of the dream state. The soul experiences pleasure and pain without the presence of the body and senses. It exists in a different dimension of time and space.

FREEDOM FROM KARMA

Within this justice system, however, there exists freedom of choice. It is we, after all, who have created this karma and we are free to change it by good actions. This is the goal of Yoga, to free ourselves from all past and hidden karmas and to stop forming new ones. This is done through non-attachment and spiritual discrimination.

Karma is produced in proportion to our attachments. Activities performed with attachment register deeper impressions on the mind. For example, if you think, imagine, and entertain a thought of hurting someone you have produced karma even if you do not physically hurt that person. If you hurt someone unknowingly, you don't produce karma. We are judged more by our intentions than our actions. The mind can bind us or free us.

Spiritual discrimination gives us the awareness that I am not the doer but merely a witness, mind and body are only instruments to please the Lord. This prevents us from producing karma. Ego and the feeling of doership produce karma while selfless service and surrendering to the will of God free us from karma.

We should accept our predicaments in life with a smiling face instead of resisting them. They are the results of our previous karma and we have to endure them. We come in contact with other souls in this life in order to fulfill karmic debts. Even though they come as friends, relatives, or enemies, we should learn to love them without attachment. We should realize that our true Self never changes; we were never born and will never die. This knowledge will free us from the chain of cause and effect. Meditation is the technique by which the mind is sufficiently steadied to gain this knowledge and bring all past karmas (mental impressions) to the surface, burning them to ashes. The yogi, freed from all karmas, has no further need to do anything and, therefore, no need to seek rebirth. He becomes liberated and universal.

BENEFITS

Understanding reincarnation has many practical benefits:

1. We are never too old to attempt something new as age is no barrier, because life is continuous. We learn new spiritual lessons and grow in wisdom as we grow older.

2. No spiritual effort is ever wasted. Lord Krishna teaches that devotees on the spiritual path are

reincarnated into a pious family and a spiritual environment. They inherit good health, have a zeal for spiritual enlightenment, and continue their spiritual journey.

3. We can realize that we are responsible for everything in our life and have created our present situation. We can stop blaming our parents, society, and various situations for our problems. This realization gives deep relaxation. We also can forgive ourselves for making mistakes in the past because we realize that those mistakes were learning experiences.

4. As we become responsible we can take charge of our life and improve its quality. We stop hoping for someone else to help us and we don't expect miracles. Instead, we realize that we can create our own miracles. For example, people who want to lose weight or stop smoking are successful only when they decide to take charge of their own life. No self-improvement program will help until one takes charge and assumes responsibility for its success.

5. Belief in reincarnation removes the fear of death as we consider death to be part of our total life. It can be thought of as a long night for the soul to rest. Like night and day, death and life cycles go on naturally. There is no fear.

6. It gives us understanding that there is no escape. Drugs, alcohol, etc. allow you to hide from the fact of life only temporarily. Suicide is not an escape as life will not end nor will it improve until we improve it ourselves.

7. We learn to be aware of our thoughts, words, and deeds because we realize that with each thought we are producing karma - positive or negative. We should channel our thoughts in a positive direction, avoiding negative thought patterns. These thoughts will become reality in time. We should learn to perform good deeds without becoming discouraged because no one can take away our reward. What we earn will come to us, and we should prevent producing bad karmas because we cannot escape punishment for them.

8. We also learn to escape karma by reducing our mental attachments. By letting go of the feeling of doership and working as an instrument of God, we don't register karma in the

memory of our biocomputer. As one evolves, reincarnation is experienced as a conviction. The realization comes to us that the world is in perfect balance and completely systematic.

9. Reincarnation increases our love and tolerance for others. Each soul is at a different level of evolution and we should not expect others to be any different. We should remember that we have gone through such experiences ourselves to come to our present level of understanding. It is normal for kindergarten children to learn the alphabet, second graders to read, and high school students to write essays. The world is a school and we are students in different grades learning different lessons. We learn to see the spark of God in everyone in spite of the different human masks they are wearing.

Karmas are debts. You can pay off debts in a few large installments, or pay smaller installments over a longer period of time but with greater interest. Adversities in life are paying off karmic debts.

Spirituality is standing on your own feet. Our feet should be firmly grounded on the earth with our experiences and convictions. Reciting someone else's ideas and philosophies is impressive to show off our knowledge, but this is not useful if it is recited like a parrot. Be thine own light.

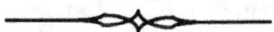

Learn to be a disciple and you will find a Guru. When a disciple is ready the Guru appears. The ocean has plenty of water, you need a container to hold its water. Make sure that the container does not have any holes and is emptied of its contents. You may not recognize a master in front of you until you open up and deserve him.

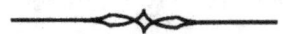

17

KARMA YOGA

The goal of Yoga is liberation or unity with higher consciousness. The different branches of Yoga lead to the same goal. These branches are: Gnana (Knowledge), Bhakti (Devotion), Karma (Action), and Raja (Mental control through meditation). One cannot practice only one form of Yoga and neglect the others. All of them must be used to some extent while making one form predominant. Karma Yoga can ideally be practiced by the average person (a householder) who is involved in worldly activities. He does not have to sacrifice any activities, go into seclusion, or practice the austerities of an ascetic. Merely by changing one's mental attitude the final goal of Yoga may be reached. Peace of mind is proportionate to the extent of practice.

THE PATH OF KARMA YOGA

Karma Yoga as described in the Bhagavad Gita could be summarized as follows: Do your duty well, wholeheartedly with love and interest. Do not let reward be the motivation for your actions. Remove the attachments of your senses so you may find peace within yourself at every moment of your life, then every action you perform will be holy. Expect no reward for your action but, at the same time, do not remain lazy or inactive because you want no reward. Rather, do all your duties selflessly and as devotion to God. This simple philosophy has tremendous potential for the individual and can help in solving many problems of life. Let us examine some of the implications of this philosophy in individual and social situations. Those who are fully absorbed in their work without thinking or worrying about the consequences put all their energy into the task at hand. Naturally, they do a better job than those who drain their energy thinking and worrying about reward. Many people believe that working or engaging in a certain activity will bring them happiness, peace, and satisfaction. They expend a great deal of energy striving for these goals. The achievement, however, is only a moment's pleasure and as it does not bring lasting satisfaction, they will then run after something else. Thus life consists of chasing after happiness which is like chasing a mirage. Real happiness is attained when one stops chasing and becomes contented. This contentment may come by absorbing one's self totally into the action being performed. For a Karma Yogi, actions in themselves are the rewards of action. Most people waste their time during week days by anticipating the weekends; a Karma Yogi enjoys both equally well.

The Law of Nature indicates that whatever goes up must come down. At the end of pleasure, pain follows. The more intense the pleasure, the more intense the pain. This is called duality (maya), for pain is hidden within pleasure itself. Karma Yoga practice allows one to transcend the dualistic mind and to experience the state of joy which flows continuously.

THE REWARDS OF KARMA YOGA

Each person is looking for freedom and happiness by employing various means and methods. Some try to find it in eating, some in sexual pleasures, others try by gaining power. The climax of their pleasure lasts for a moment and then tapers off. If we examine this moment, our so-called pleasure is nothing but a state of loss. At this moment one loses his own self and lets go completely with no inhibitions. Karma Yoga uses the technique of losing ourselves in the action being performed regardless of what that action is. If one loses himself in washing dishes or serving others in some capacity, one experiences a state of constant joy. This is true freedom because you do not rely on anything external for producing this happiness; you are the master of all situations.

Karma Yoga practice matures one and provides freedom from petty emotions. These petty emotions can make man a servant and compel him to be excited or depressed beyond his control. Inner peace comes when one is free from these emotions. The boat without an engine is pushed around by the current and the wind. The boat with an engine is not at their mercy. Karma Yoga makes one strong and independent like the boat with an engine.

When work is performed for its own sake, without seeking any reward, there are no tensions and work becomes play. The difference between work and play lies within one's mental attitude. Games are fun all of the time regardless of winning or losing. Unfortunately competition is so deeply engraved in our minds that we cannot even play a game for the game's sake. We go bowling or golfing, setting goals for ourselves and producing tension instead of relaxation. Yoga says if you perform all your actions with love and interest your work will become play.

KARMA YOGA AND DUTY (DHARMA)

How can one determine one's own duty? Standards of duty vary from nation to nation, from culture to culture. There are many duties which are born of nature. One has duty towards himself, his family, neighbors, and society. The best guide for determining one's duty is one's own conscience. One must purify himself through Yamas and Niyamas (See Chapter 3.) the moral code of conduct in Yoga, so that one develops a clear conscience which will respond to the questions of duty. The duties of everyone are described in Hindu and Yogic scriptures and will be discussed later. These duties are so universal and uniquely set forth that, with slight adaptations, they could apply to all religions, cultures, and types of environment.

Many people ask the question: How can you work if you have no goal? The answer is that one must have a goal, one must determine the direction in which he wants to go. Once that direction is determined, however, you don't have to think of how far you are from the final goal or become anxious about it. This thought will make you aware of time and produce anxiety and tension. For example, if you are traveling from Philadelphia to New York, you get on the highway which leads there, but if it takes three hours you do not continually think of the time. You go in the proper direction, keeping your eyes on the road and acting in the present. You may use crossroads and other landmarks to assure that you are on the right path. However, if you say you should be in New York within three hours and should not encounter any traffic, then you are not practicing Karma Yoga because you are caught up in expecting the results of your actions. Also, the constant thought of the future may distract you from the present moment, causing you to miss a turn or an exit, or cause an accident due to absent mindedness.

Some people say that they like to think of the past or derive pleasure by thinking about a future event rather than enjoying the present moment. This attitude keeps people asleep. They cannot hear, see, or experience anything new. Those who wait for a party all day long, begin worrying about going home when the party begins. Karma Yoga teaches one to live in the present and to be aware. Experiencing is living and growing. Living through imagination of the past or the future is like being dead while alive. If you go on vacation and spend your time taking pictures for the memory of it and to impress your friends, you miss the real experience of being there.

If you perform your duties with no thought of gain, you may receive a better reward. Should you give up this reward? No. Accept it without likes or dislikes. A good reward should not excite you; poor results should not make you unhappy. This is the state of the lotus flower on the lake. It lives in the water, yet water does not touch it. This is the true state of yogic non-attachment.

The Karma Yogi has to work constantly. There is no failure for him. Since he does not get depressed by failure, he tries again until the final goal is reached. Each moment is fresh and new. Ultimately one understands the secret of work and sees that it is not done by him but by Prakriti, divine energy flowing through him. The realization comes that I am not the doer. That is the true freedom of the Karma Yogi.

The Yogic Theory of Karma teaches that everyone is bound by the laws of karma (the laws of cause and effect). Good karma brings rewards and bad karma brings suffering. Each action produces karma, and the goal of Yoga is to be free from all karmas and to reach final liberation. When the Karma Yogi performs his actions without any attachment, he does not produce any karma and evolves faster on the path of Yoga.

SCRIPTURAL AUTHORITY

In Hinduism there are scriptures from Vedic times dating back six thousand years which describe the many duties of men and women, be they kings, queens, employers, or employees, giving them guidance on the path of Karma Yoga. This guidance is very practical even today. One should keep the central idea in mind and apply it to his personal life in the best possible way. These scriptures are entitled Manu Smruti Sutras and Gruhya Sutras. They have influenced Indian culture all these years and have been found to be very effective. In more recent years degradation took place as people followed these scriptural teachings as social customs without understanding them in their true spirit.

There are four caste systems: 1. Brahmins (priests and spiritual guides), 2. Kshatriya (warriors or protectors of society), 3. Vaishya (business class who take care of the welfare of society), and 4. Shudra (servant class who take care of the utilities of society). Westerners criticize this caste system because they have seen only the misuse and negative side of it.

The central idea of the caste system is that one's duty is determined from birth which makes it easier to concentrate on that profession, and the trade can go from father to child. One chooses a particular family, caste, parents, environment, and talents according to one's spiritual evolution. One should accept such natural situations in life as one's own dharma. It is said in the Gita that your own dharma (duty) done properly is superior to someone else's duty. A servant may reach the final goal of Yoga by doing his duty well, although it is socially inferior to the duties of a Brahmin. In today's society one's dharma is unclear and the work needed to satisfy the individual soul is obscured. In your own environment you may determine your own duty. If you are a teacher or priest, you call yourself Brahmin. If you perform any type of service for society, you are a Shudra. Yoga also describes four stages (Ashrams) of life: 1. Student, 2. Householder, 3. Anchorite, and 4. Ascetic. Performing these duties at their proper time is one's dharma. Scriptures describe four attainments in life: 1. Artha (prosperity), 2. Kama (pleasure), 3. Dharma (spiritual life), and 4. Moksha (Liberation). One should fulfill prosperity and pleasure through spiritual means and yearn for liberation as the ultimate goal in life.

JOINT FAMILY SYSTEM

The strength of a piece of cloth is determined by the strength of the individual threads. Each family is an important unit of society. The real strength of society lies in its moral and spiritual solidity, without which the political and material strength crumble. Peace and harmony in the individual family bring peace and harmony to the nation. These days we see the social trend of families disintegrating and turning into broken or single parent families. There is a mass of people but no society. In some instances the only thing that keeps them together is the law and this is compulsion, not free will or love.

Yoga practices start from your own self. First we must find harmony within ourselves, then with our family, then relatives, friends, neighbors, etc. We must face reality and not run away from it.

Psychologically, it has been surveyed and proven that people engrossed in the family are happier than the loners. Even insurance companies consider loners to be poor risks; most criminals are loners.

In the joint family parents and children live in unity with each other. Many times several generations live under the same roof, sharing their income along with good and bad times. The elders are respected and their advice sought by others. Parents support their children until they complete their schooling. A real sense of love and responsibility ties everyone together. All the earnings go in the same pot and are shared according to needs. In the absence of the father, the oldest son becomes responsible for the family. The parents are worshiped and in their old age the sons and daughters take care of them.

The goal of Yoga is to remove or reduce the lower ego. In the joint family the children learn we and us, not I and mine. Older members take care of the younger ones. Shared experiences and materials provide fulfillment and keep everyone together. To whatever extent one removes I and mine, to that extent consciousness expands. In childhood these seeds of selflessness are sown very easily. One learns the lesson that true freedom is born out of responsibility and mastery of self. The opportunity to fully develop individuality through the nurturing of selfless love, service, and patience is present in the joint family system. One learns that temporary pleasures and material gain do not bring true happiness or inner tranquility.

In the West personal independence is over-emphasized. For example, after marriage the children seldom maintain close ties with their parents. This independence can become intolerance if one becomes used to selfish ways and cannot tolerate another person's views or habits. In the joint family one learns acceptance and how to make necessary adjustments to be contented in life. One learns to share the material, emotional, and spiritual aspects of life.

Joy is doubled when it is shared and sorrows are reduced when shared by all family members. When there is sharing in the family there is no need for a psychiatrist, a word hardly known in close families. When there is no family closeness one joins clubs and organizations to alleviate loneliness, or pays a psychiatrist to talk to him.

It is human nature to seek out companions and to share. An unhappy family life forces the youngster to run away from his parents and to join the commune family. Going to a commune may be an escape from reality and its responsibilities. One learns unconditional love in the joint family which is then extended to friends. For example, when eating out, the one who has the money treats others to a meal with no expectation of a return. Accepting favors from each other brings each person closer to this unconditional love. One feels free to talk about personal matters and this releases mental pressure.

On trains and buses in India, you hear strangers talking of personal matters such as family income or about their children and their problems. People feel free to offer advice and comfort. With this openness of heart one does not need group therapy. When there is a problem with any member of society, neighbors and strangers rush to help. In the West people do not want to get involved. Sometimes they don't know who their next door neighbor is. Many crimes take place because people are engrossed in themselves and are not involved in mutual matters. At the scene of a murder, robbery, rape, or car accident, they run away to avoid involvement instead of running to offer help.

SOCIETY

In addition to the family, one has his duties towards society. One may be employed as a secretary, a mechanic, a nurse, or may be self-employed. If one does his duty well, it indirectly influences society in the form of better services, better products, and better morale. The general trend in the West is less work for more pay, resulting in strikes and salary raises which then raise the price of the products. Overall services and quality of products are getting poorer. This can be verified by people who have gone to the emergency ward of a hospital, taken their car for service, or have had experience with utility services, doctors, or lawyers.

Although there is more prosperity than ever before, crimes are increasing in spite of more efficient locks, alarms, and well trained dogs in many homes. Insurance coverage is continually on the increase. Still people feel insecure and are afraid to walk the streets at night. Real security comes from inner peace. If every one practices his dharma wholeheartedly and with love there will be peace at the personal level which eventually will bring about political, economic, and social transformation.

When there is a strong society, social customs control the conduct of the people. When there is a weak society conduct is left to the laws, but as more laws are established more loopholes are found to escape them. Laws govern our lives rather than moral conduct and understanding. There are many unnecessary court hearings, disturbances, and complications which distract one from his basic goal and aim in life. We need only food and shelter for living which should be a simple matter, but we get caught by the complications of self-made slavery.

MARRIAGE

Karma Yoga is very important in a marriage relationship. Women are naturally feminine; their gentleness, love, and emotional qualities balance and complement the innate reasoning, toughness, and aggressiveness of men. Eastern scriptures say that a woman's duty is to her parents when she is young and to her husband and children after marriage. A man's duty is to provide for the welfare and protection of his family.

In the East marriage is prearranged. Parents and relatives match the bride and groom by considering family backgrounds, culture, education, wealth, social status, and astrological charts, as well as approval of the prospective parties. The betrothal (engagement) increases family ties as the bride and groom are invited for dinner at each other's house. Dating is not permitted, but they may see each other and talk in the presence of an escort. They are later united in marriage with such elaborate rituals that the ceremony is a memorable event, not only for them but also for the whole town. Love grows after marriage and they accept each other for the rest of their lives for whatever they are and make the necessary adjustments. In this way, marriage can act as a basis for mutual spiritual growth and as a framework for selfless service, love, contentment, and humility.

Western style marriage encourages first love then marriage. Two strangers meet and are attracted towards each other. Even after dating for years they remain strangers because in their attraction they can see only the positive side of the partner. After some time this attraction wears off and they face reality, seeing their partner in his or her true spirit. If expectations are high, they may start seeing the faults of their partner which leads to disharmony and possibly separation, adultery, or divorce. Jealousy, fear, and an overemphasis on sensual attachments keep the mind and emotions in a turmoil. When one is permitted many partners he comes to know them only superficially, which results in more exposure and experience before marriage and makes marriage itself an ordinary event instead of a lifetime commitment. One has a hard time committing himself to a single person and getting beyond the level of superficial pleasures.

Freedom is like a knife. It can be used constructively or destructively. Social freedom allows the use of mental freedom. Should a quarrel or problem arise between a couple, they think of the possibility of separation or divorce. If, however, separation or divorce is made extremely difficult, they might try to work it out. When one has freedom from elders and society, one easily finds fault with his spouse and may become attracted to a new person.

Occasions like marriage, joyous holidays, or sickness and death which require the gathering of relatives, encourage closeness and communication. The ability to gather with family members and to communicate with them makes working out marriage problems much easier. The purpose of marriage must not be limited to sensual gratification, but should include disciplining, harmonizing, and letting love grow into spiritual love. Husband and wife are considered to be two wheels of a chariot and they must work together to make life's journey smooth. The duty of husband and wife towards each other should be considered holy. The householder doing his duties has the same potential for spiritual evolution as the ascetic who has renounced the world in search of God.

Harmony is a very important aspect of marriage. Husband and wife eventually lose much of their individual identity and become one. There should be no secrets between them, such as a separate bank account. Ideally women should stay home to take proper care of the children, especially when they are very young. Children should accompany their parents on as many occasions as possible as they find satisfaction and love by being with them and sharing experiences. It has been found that children who don't receive their parents' love when they are young suffer from psychological problems when they are older. Not enough time spent with children is a major cause of the generation gap today. Children learn the best lessons of their lives by watching their parents and by staying with them, rather than hearing them preach. The harmony of the parents helps in the growth of the children. Activities should be done together when possible. If husband and wife take an interest in each other's activities or do them together, this will provide moral support and encouragement for spiritual evolution. Working parents have very little time to spend on mutual activities which are necessary to maintain harmony and unity.

The practice of Karma Yoga should gradually develop into service for all humanity so that eventually one sees God in all human beings and ultimately in all living creatures. It should develop to the extent that one does not see himself as being different from others. In the real sense no one can help anyone else; we should consider service an opportunity for our own growth. The world is full of good and evil and it will remain that way as long as it exists. It may be helpful to think of the world as a laboratory and Karma Yoga as the technique to evolve to the final goal of Self-realization.

Transform your personality from inside out. When you build the center inside, let the outside be projected naturally. Don't pretend to love someone, smile and act happy on the surface while you have anger, fear, and resentment inside. Do not suppress negative emotions, release them in a constructive manner. If you heal a wound on the surface while the inside is infected, it will only increase internal infection with greater intensity.

Use hugs and touching with your family members. Hugging and touching unite prana and healing energy thus dissolving all barriers of communication. Love and hugs can provide energy to young infants and patients in nursing homes. Life is sustained by love. Life thrives on love. Material gifts and flowery speech are not substitutes for a warm hug or touch.

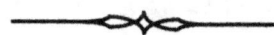

Karma Yoga

It is a matter of habit to see any situation in a positive or negative way. A cup is half-full or half-empty depending upon our perception. We are conditioned to likes and dislikes. We can learn to appreciate cloudy weather and rain as much as sunny weather. We have to be aware and look at the beauty in each situation and environment.

**

Don't entertain any negative thought for a prolonged period of time. Dwelling on it and creating an image in the mind may turn it into reality. We have full choice of projecting our own reality. Some people project failure, rejection, accidents, etc. Others project success, love, and good fortune.

**

Results of meditation are gradual. Patience is required. Progress is subtle like a growing child. Don't give up practice if you can't see tangible results immediately. Do not uproot a plant or ignore it if it does not bear fruit immediately.

**

We have limited time in a day. If you want to accomplish something, set priorities.

**

Fanatics have rigid blind faith. _Eccentrics_ have one-pointed energy - mostly misdirected. _Skeptics_ reject faith and close themselves to experiences. _Fatalists_ escape reality out of fear and accept things inactively, yet hoping for a reward by some miracle. The _Man of Wisdom_ has an open mind, open heart and dynamic faith, and performs his duties to please the Lord.

**

A camel was complaining about the crooked tail of a dog, crooked beak of a parrot, crooked neck of a stork, and the crooked tusks of an elephant. When he looked into the mirror he found that he had crooked limbs himself. We should do introspection in order to work on our own problems and faults instead of criticizing others. We don't see our faults and often magnify the small faults of others.

****

DIET

18. Diet and Nutrition

19. Yoga and Diet

20. Natural and Health Foods

21. Vegetarianism

22. Fasting

23. Cleansing

24. Vegetarian Recipes

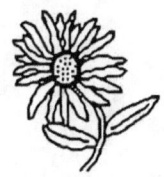

18

DIET AND NUTRITION

INTRODUCTION TO DIET

Some people eat only to live. They are generally unaware of their eating habits and don't really enjoy their food; for them eating is a burden. There are others who live only to eat. Although they certainly enjoy their food, they have little or no regard for its nutritional value or the quantity, thus jeopardizing their health. Chapter 24 offers balanced recipes that insure pleasurable eating as well as proper nourishment.

Efficient digestion of any food depends largely upon the mental preparation for eating it. Appearance and odor play important roles in digestion. Many of the herbs and spices which we use stimulate the appetite thereby increasing the secretion of digestive juices and enzymes. They are also marvelous remedies for many health problems as well as serving as preservatives when no refrigeration is available.

Practitioners of Yoga develop a natural desire to avoid meat and they usually assume a vegetarian diet. They are often held back due to lack of information on its ease and practicality. Westerners who are used to eating meat, poultry, and seafood all their lives cannot imagine how it is possible to abstain from eating meat. They imagine a vegetarian diet to be bland and uninteresting, consisting only of salads and vegetables. The Hindu culture has been vegetarian for thousands of years and has developed menus that would amaze the meat eating world. They can prepare beans, grains, vegetables, and fruits in hundreds of varied ways.

Many people who are concerned about getting proper nourishment have the idea that if you do not eat meat you will not receive enough protein. This is not true. Soya beans, for instance, contain more protein than meat. Also, the proper combination of beans and grains will provide essential amino acids.

Vegetarians are the healthiest people in the world. Many diseases common to meat eating countries are unknown to vegetarian countries. The reason for people being unhealthy in these vegetarian countries is not due to vegetarianism, but rather it is due to the fact that they do not have enough food to provide them with a properly balanced diet. As you explore the possibilities offered in this and the following chapters, your craving for meat will decrease.

NUTRITION

To maintain good health we need a diet that provides balanced nutrition. Such a diet would include proteins, carbohydrates, fats, vitamins, minerals, enzymes, and water. A vegetarian diet is perfect for providing all of these nutrients.

PROTEINS Protein molecules are made of carbon, hydrogen, oxygen, and nitrogen. Combinations of several amino acids make up these protein molecules. There are eight amino acids derived from food which are called essential amino acids. Other amino acids are manufactured in the digestive canal. Many amino acids are available at health food stores in free form, individually or in combination. They are excellent for metabolizing fat, losing weight, dissolving cholesterol, or for neuronutrition. Vegetarians can find complete protein by eating brown rice and bean soup, or cornbread and beans as a staple diet. Protein is needed for growth and proper functioning of the body. Milk, cheese, eggs, nuts, beans, flours, and brewer's yeast are good sources of protein.

CARBOHYDRATES Carbohydrates are made up of carbon, hydrogen, and oxygen. Carbohydrates provide our body with the principle energy. They can be obtained in the form of simple or complex sugars. Starches break down into glucose and are digested in the small intestine. Excess glucose is stored in the liver in the form of glycogen for future use. Some starches are stored in the form of fat throughout the body. Most foods contain some simple carbohydrates. We do not need to eat any refined sugar. Honey, sweet fruits, dried fruits, etc. contain simple sugars while grains and legumes contain complex sugars.

FATS Fats are a concentrated food and take a long time to digest. Secretion of bile from the gall bladder softens it, enzymes of the pancreas break it down, and the intestines absorb it. Some fat is stored in the liver, but most is stored in the inactive parts of the body.

Fats are available in saturated and unsaturated forms. Unsaturated fats are easy to digest and are more beneficial than saturated fats. Milk, butter, oil from corn, sunflower, sesame, soya, peanut, olive, etc. are good suppliers of fats.

VITAMINS and MINERALS Vitamins and minerals are needed for our body to remain healthy. Minerals are like bricks and vitamins are like mortar. Both are required in combination for effective utilization.

Vitamins: VITAMIN A builds resistance to infection and prevents night blindness. Lack of this vitamin causes many problems like retarded growth, dry skin, poor vision, and hair problems. It is found in tomatoes, raw carrots, spinach, buttermilk, eggs, and green and yellow vegetables and fruits.

VITAMIN B-COMPLEX is a group of many B vitamins, thiamin, riboflavin, pyridoxine, niacin, B-12, and many other vitamins. They are needed for normal growth of the body and for the nerves. Fresh vegetables, eggs, milk, cheese, beans, and whole grains contain vitamin B-complex.

VITAMIN C controls oxidation processes in the body. It is required for healthy blood vessels and teeth. It is also a good cleanser and is helpful in avoiding or curing colds. Vitamin C is found in green leafy vegetables, citrus fruits, tomatoes, beans, sprouts, and raw carrots.

VITAMIN D is needed for healthy bones and teeth and is found in milk, cream, eggs, and the sun's rays.

One should eat a variety of fruits and vegetables to ensure that all required vitamins are available in the daily diet. Some are effective only in combination with others. Our earth is depleted of some nutrients and one cannot be sure of getting all the vitamins and minerals through food even if one eats properly. It is recommended that one take a superior quality natural one-a-day vitamin which contains the necessary vitamins, minerals, and trace minerals. These are available at health food stores.

One may need additional vitamins for specific needs. Vegetarians should take a good B-complex vitamin containing the eight essential amino acids which the body does not manufacture.

One should take vitamins with the major meal of the day so they can be utilized properly. Vitamins A, D, E, and K are fat soluble while the others are water soluble. Vitamins

Diet and Nutrition

should be taken in time release form so the body obtains steady nutrition over a period of time. Also, minerals should be taken in orotate or chelated form as the body utilizes them more efficiently than regular minerals.

Megavitamin dosage is only recommended for a limited time for helping specific ailments. This should be done under the guidance of a nutritionist.

Minerals: Minerals can only be used by the body if they are organic. Many processed foods turn organic molecules into inorganic molecules which cannot be utilized by the body. Calcium, magnesium, phosphorous, iron, iodine, copper, sodium, potassium, chlorine, manganese, fluorine, zinc, selenium, chromium, and trace minerals, etc. are required by the body.

CALCIUM builds bones and teeth, and is part of nerve and muscle tissue. Vegetables, nuts, milk, cheese, and eggs are good sources of calcium. Calcium should be taken with magnesium in a 2:1 ratio of Ca/Mg in order to utilize the calcium.

IRON helps the blood carry oxygen. Green vegetables, fried fruits, whole grains, lentils, peas, spinach, eggs, and cereals contain iron.

PHOSPHOROUS works with calcium in maintaining an acid base balance in the body. It also builds bones and teeth. Foods containing calcium also contain phosphorous.

IODINE regulates the thyroid gland which governs the body's use of energy. Iodized table salt, berries, pineapple, garlic, spinach, beets, pears, and mushrooms are some foods containing iodine.

CHLORINE is a good cleanser for the body. Leafy greens, table salt, milk, beets, etc. contain chlorine.

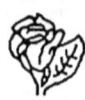

Prayer should be active. Prayer gives inspiration and guidance that should be utilized. In a flood a devotee prayed, God sent him a boat and then a helicopter but he did not accept them and he drowned.

ACID-ALKALINE BALANCING

Proper balance of acidic and alkaline foods should be consumed to maintain body chemistry. When animal starches and proteins are metabolized they produce uric, sulfuric, and phosphoric acids. These form an acidic ash as residue.

As fruits and vegetables metabolize they form salts of alkalizing metals like calcium, magnesium, sodium, and potassium. Most acid fruits such as oranges and grapefruit also produce an alkaline ash. Dairy products and vegetable oils produce a neutral residue.

A balanced diet should contain 80% alkalizing food and 20% acid forming food. Alkalizing substances should remain in reserve to neutralize acid forming foods. Over-acidity in body tissues causes many problems, such as arthritis, rheumatic disorders, etc. Most common foods are acidic. One should eat plenty of fruits and vegetables in order to maintain this balance. Caffeine, sugar, flours, meat, fish, processed foods, drugs, soft drinks, and ice cream are examples of acid forming foods and should be eaten sparingly or not at all.

Stress does not come from outside. It is our reactions to situations that produce stress. There are healthy stresses which keep our energy active and functioning properly. Unhealthy stress comes when our mind over-reacts to situations. The mind wants to finish a whole year's work in one day. Live one hour at a time.

When one is not centered one has no direction. Society and various situations push him around like a dry leaf pushed by the wind. A balanced and centered person is like fruit coming straight down from the tree due to its own weight.

19

YOGA AND DIET

We are made up of what we eat. Mind is the finer product of the body so not only our physical but also our mental development depend upon the kind of food we eat. In the Bhagavad Gita, the ancient scriptures of Yoga, the three qualities of food are described as the gunas. They are: 1. Satvik or pure, 2. Rajasik or stimulating, and 3. Tamasik or promoting inertia. A person's mental qualities depend upon the kind of food he eats, and the kind of food someone desires depends upon his mental growth and preparation. As one evolves spiritually the Tamasik qualities should be reduced as the Satvik qualities increase.

SATVIK FOOD (Pure Food)

Satvik food helps promote purity and calmness of mind, awareness of our higher being, and peace of mind. Mental concentration and contentment increase, and feelings of lightness and alertness appear. Satvik food gives the body proper nourishment and helps dispense with restlessness, tension, and other mental disturbances.

Fresh fruits and vegetables, milk, butter and other dairy products, nuts and grains, and dry fruits are all Satvik foods. Their taste is pleasant and sweet.

RAJASIK FOOD (Stimulating Food)

Rajasik food produces restlessness of the body and mind because of its stimulating effect on the nervous system. Rajasik food tends to increase desire, passion, hatred, restlessness, and hunger. Meat, alcohol, fish, eggs, and hot and spicy foods are in this category. Their taste is salty and pungent.

TAMASIK FOOD (Impure, Contaminated Food)

Tamasik food produces inertia, dullness, slothfulness, laziness, etc. One lacks energy and awareness of material or spiritual life. Living like animals with no motivation or purpose in life is very common, as is suffering from chronic diseases like heart problems, constipation, sluggishness, and breathing disturbances. Contaminated, rotten, putrefied, overripe, stale, and leftover food come under this category. Tamasik food is bitter and tasteless.

PRANA

According to Yoga the entire universe is made of akash and prana. Akash is matter and prana is the unit of energy behind all the movements and activities in the universe. When prana leaves the body the person is pronounced dead. Prana exists in our body in the form of heart and lung movement, brain activity, and activity of the cells and body tissues. The body receives prana from food, drink, breath, sleep, and sunshine.

Food is one of the important mediums for receiving prana. Advanced yogis can receive prana directly from the air or through the atmosphere and can sustain life with a minimal amount of food. Prana is stored in the solar plexus located below the navel. People with a greater amount of prana radiate it in the form of health, vitality, cheerfulness, optimism, and contentment. In addition, they have greater concentration and clairvoyance. Their presence is soothing and comforting, and their speech is sweet and effective. Those who lack sufficient prana also lack the above qualities. Since food is one of the principle sources of prana and we eat three times a day, it makes a considerable difference what and how we eat.

In Yoga the body is considered to be the temple of God. God would not want to live in an unclean place. The body is the most important instrument a man has for perceiving God. It must be purified and made healthy. If the body is not healthy the mind will not be healthy. A man who does not feel well physically cannot sit restfully, think properly or concentrate, and will not be successful in life. To perceive God one has to control the mind, and mind cannot be controlled without first controlling the body. The food we eat determines our physical health, but most people are too concerned about the pleasure of eating and pay little attention to important dietary rules. Yoga recommends the following points:

DIET RECOMMENDATIONS

1. CHEWING WELL. Chewing strengthens the gums and provides good exercise. It increases secretion of enzymes which helps with digestion. When food is softened and turned into liquid form the stomach uses less energy in digestion. Chewing allows enough time for the nerve impulse to reach the

brain and one becomes satisfied with less food. Also, chewing well prevents one from overeating.

2. EAT ONLY WHEN HUNGRY AND DO NOT OVEREAT. By instinct animals do not eat when they are sick or not hungry. Humans, being superior to animals, have a conscious mind which may be used constructively or destructively. Humans eat to satisfy their desire for taste even when they are not hungry and this habit reduces their life span. If food is put into the stomach beyond its digestive capacity or when we are not hungry, it remains stagnant and the organs of digestion and elimination as well as the heart must work harder to direct the food into the proper channels.

Overeating and eating without hunger reduce the digestive capacity of the stomach causing sluggishness and malnutrition. Even if nourishing food is eaten along with worthless food, the nourishing food does not digest properly. If the organs are continually overworked their life span decreases. Accumulated waste in the various organs increases the residue and toxicity of the body and the residual food in the intestines becomes fermented causing constipation and many diseases.

As we grow older our body's metabolism slows down, the construction process in the body slows, and deterioration begins. At this time if a person concentrates on eating less than his hunger calls for and eats only one or two meals a day, he will reduce the degeneration of the body and live a longer and healthier life.

Yoga recommends undereating. Fill the stomach halfway, leave one-fourth room for water and one-fourth for air. This keeps the digestive fire alive. When coal is added a little bit at a time to a charcoal grill the fire grows strong. If the fire is covered completely with charcoal it dies. In the same way, if we keep our digestive fire alive we develop resistance and immunity against infections. When our digestive fire is reduced we become susceptible to colds and infections.

Yogis say that our life span is measured by the number of breaths not by the number of years. Overeating shortens our breath and increases the rate of breathing. When the diet is light, breathing is deep and rhythmic which makes it easier for the mind to be calm and peaceful. A full stomach requires a great deal of blood circulation for digestion which leaves the brain starving for blood. This reduces mental alertness, promotes laziness, and contributes to a premature death.

3. SCHEDULE REGULAR MEALS. Avoid eating between meals as this spoils the appetite. If meals are scheduled at a regular time our stomach will secrete digestive juices at those times and digestion will be complete. Even eating a small piece of cake, a cooky, candy, or a few peanuts between meals will start secretion of digestive juices and hunger will be reduced at the next meal. An irregular schedule causes irregularity in elimination resulting in constipation problems. Schedule a weekly fasting day. This will form a regular rhythm and your body will be ready for the fast making it a natural and effortless process. (See Chapter 22 for details on fasting.)

4. EMOTIONAL STATE OF MIND. Our stomach and digestive organs are closely connected with our nervous system. Our internal organs, especially our stomach, function properly only when our mind is calm and relaxed. When the mind is excited, depressed, or worried real hunger is killed. If food is put into the stomach at this time it remains dormant and causes many problems. Try to avoid eating when angry, excited, sick, tired, depressed, hurried, or worried. It is like poisoning the stomach to eat at these times. Wait until the mind calms down and hunger returns.

Always eat in pleasant surroundings and in a peaceful mood. Persons with a calm mind burn less energy and require less nutrition for a healthy life. People with restless minds suffer from deficiencies in spite of a nutritious diet. It is a sad thing to observe employees gulping their food during a short lunch break and executives, who have enough time to eat properly, being involved in serious business talks or arguments while eating. Talking and eating do not complement each other.

Yoga teaches that we should first pray to God for being fortunate enough to have the meal. Accept the food as Prasad (Mercy of God). Be aware of what you are eating and the process of eating. Visualize the process of digestion and feel the food being converted into the life energy, prana. Eating with awareness increases discipline in eating habits and makes us think of our stomach as a sacred place before putting burdens into it.

5. AVOID PROCESSED AND CANNED FOODS. Many kinds of foods are prepared for profit rather than for health. Preservatives and chemicals, which are harmful to our health, are added to increase the shelf life of the food. The bad effects of these may be seen soon or they may not be seen for another generation. Many foods available today are processed

and essential parts of the original wholesome food have been separated leaving only such things as refined starch, while the nutritious part is fed to farm animals. White bread and refined sugar are examples of this.

When food is canned it is heated at high temperatures to destroy microbes and this destroys many of the natural nutrients along with the microbes. Protein does survive high temperatures but it loses its regenerating and rebuilding qualities.

6. DRINK PLENTY OF WATER. Water is an excellent body cleanser. If you drink slightly warm water on arising it will help eliminate constipation problems. During the night and at the last stages of digestion most of the moisture is absorbed in the large intestine leaving the waste dry and causing constipation. Warm water helps loosen waste and improve elimination within a few minutes after drinking. During the day drink 5 to 8 glasses of water to flush the system and remove toxins. Avoid drinking cold water as this reduces the digestive capacity. Do not drink water with meals as this dilutes the digestive juices. Always drink water slowly. Most city water contains inorganic ions which are not good for our systems. The water in vegetables has organic ions which our body can utilize. Therefore, you should drink the water in which vegetables are cooked or steamed. City and well water can be contaminated with harmful chemicals. Use a reliable water filter to remove harmful contaminants. Spring water is ideal for everyday use and it provides important minerals for the body, but be sure it is obtained from a reliable source. Distilled water contains no minerals but is ideal to use during fasting and cleansing. Regular use of distilled water will extract important minerals from the body. Take an orotate or chelated mineral supplement if you plan to use distilled water for a prolonged period.

7. AVOID SWEETS, STIMULANTS, AND DRUGS. Candy, ice cream, and most other sweets supply useless calories without nutrition as they contain refined sugar and refined flours. The craving for sweets can be satisfied by eating nutritious fresh or dried fruits. Tea, coffee, soda, and other stimulants should be avoided. Caffeine and tannic acid increase insulin production in the blood stream temporarily producing an energy increase, but they leave you depressed later on. The use of stimulants also reduces the appetite, weakens digestion, and is habit forming.

Alcohol and smoking are prohibited for the Yoga practitioner. Alcohol destroys vitamin B-complex and produces mental dullness. Smoking produces a vitamin C deficiency and lung diseases. Avoid the use of prescription drugs as much as possible. They lower the natural resistance of the body, often produce side effects, and they stay in the body for extended periods. If you must take antibiotics you should take an acidophilus supplement to replace the friendly bacteria in the intestines.

When the body is attuned to balanced nourishment and the functions of the inner organs are normalized, the desire for wrong foods and stimulants disappears. Yoga is the process of mastery of the Self. Slavery to any habits, especially bad habits, is to be avoided.

8. FOOD AS MEDIUM FOR THOUGHTS.

Yogis eat at home as much as possible. The thoughts and vibrations of the person preparing the food are transmitted to the one who eats it. For this reason Hindu custom does not allow a person of the higher caste to eat or drink anything at the house of a person of a lower caste. It is very important for a person to be careful where he eats when he is trying to practice spiritual disciplines. To one who has no goal it makes no difference. Also, advanced masters won't be affected by the lower vibrations. If a saintly person eats for a while at the house of a sinner he is likely to be converted into a sinner in time. If a sinner dines at the house of a saint he is likely to acquire the qualities of the saint.

Wives can uplift their husbands and children if they chant mantras while cooking. Mothers in India chant mantras while cooking and this produces harmony in the entire family through the secret ingredient of love which they put into their meals.

9. AVOID WRONG COMBINATIONS.

Animals maintain a simple diet and eat only one kind of food at a time. Humans combine many kinds of food at one meal and this is responsible for much of the indigestion and gas problems. The process of digestion means the breakdown of food particles and absorption of them into our blood stream. Enzymes act as a catalyst and play a very important role in digestion. Many enzymes are specific in their activities and we know that protein, carbohydrates, and fats are digested by specific enzymes. The kind of enzyme secreted depends upon the kind of food eaten, and when only one kind of food is eaten the enzymes are strong enough to digest that food effectively. When several categories of foods are eaten together the enzymes become modified and consequently leave some food undigested. The combination of acidic and alkaline enzymes neutralize one another. This combination results in a reduction of the digestive capacity.

The wrong combination changes the timing of enzyme secretion and food that could digest in a short time if taken alone, will stay undigested for a longer time when in combination with certain other foods. Avoid the following combinations as much as possible:

A. PROTEIN AND STARCH: This combination is widely used in sandwiches or when meat is combined with potatoes. Starches digest in the mouth with alkaline enzymes, while protein digests in the stomach in an acidic medium. The combination of acids with alkali causes gas and the starch remains undigested. The correct method is to eat protein first and then starch to insure proper digestion of both.

B. ACID FRUITS AND STARCH: Do not eat grapefruit with cereals. Acid fruits destroy some enzymes which suspends digestion of starch. Eat the grapefruit at least one half hour before the rest of your breakfast.

C. PROTEIN AND PROTEIN: Eat only one concentrated protein food at a time. Do not drink milk and eat meat or eggs at the same meal. Protein combinations change the secretion time for the enzymes and digestion takes longer.

D. FAT AND PROTEIN: Avoid excessive fats and fried foods. Fats eaten with protein have an inhibiting effect on gastric juices and make protein digestion difficult. Eat some green vegetables to reduce this inhibiting effect.

E. STARCH AND SUGAR: Avoid refined sugar as much as possible. Sugar digests in the small intestine and, when combined with starch or protein, begins to ferment quickly and remains in the stomach for a longer time. Cake, pastry, etc. are good examples of this wrong combination.

Try not to eat fruits and vegetables together. Green vegetables and salads are suitable to mix with either starch or protein. Avoid the other combinations as much as possible. Eat raw foods first then the main meal. Also, milk is a food as well as a drink. Take it alone and do not drink it instead of water.

In addition, try and take only one food high in protein or starch at one meal. Many foods in their natural form contain combinations of carbohydrates, proteins, vitamins, etc. which are easy to digest. Therefore, by consuming these natural foods we do not have to be concerned about properly balanced nutrition.

Maintain a pleasant variety in your menu to insure the maximum amount of nutrition.

Wrong food combinations or overeating do not kill anyone directly but they do so indirectly and slowly. As improper digestion and elimination put extra burdens on the body, we function below our physical and mental potential. When vital energy decreases and toxicity increases, immunity and resistance decrease causing allergies, infections, and a shorter life span.

AYURVEDA

Ayu means life and Veda means knowledge. Ayurveda provides knowledge for healthy living. It is a five thousand year old science of India. The human body is made of five basic elements: Earth, Water, Air, Ether, and Fire (Samkhya Yoga). These elements combine with each other and form three basic principles (humors) called TRI DOSHA.

ELEMENT COMBINATIONS

1. Earth and Water produce Kapha Dosha, Biological Movement.
2. Water and Fire produce Pitta Dosha, Bodily Heat Energy.
3. Air and Ether produce Vata Dosha, Biological Water.

These three doshas govern all bodily functions. When they are in balance one remains healthy. Each person is born with certain genetic combinations which are composed of a mixture of tri dosha in different proportions. Food is composed of the same five elements and each food promotes certain dosha.

By understanding one's own constitution and conditions in particular situations, one can bring about proper balance and healing by balancing tri dosha with proper foods.

Yoga and Diet

20

NATURAL AND HEALTH FOODS

Many people today suffer from malnutrition and other physical deficiencies despite the fact that they eat what is considered to be a nutritious diet. Vitamins are advertised extensively as providing more than 100% of the minimum daily requirements, yet there are more problems than ever before. One answer is that our food is not wholesome. Most of the products available in the market today are commercially produced in such a way that nutritional standards become secondary to business and profit considerations.

Many foods are shipped great distances, then they are stored on the shelf. In order to keep them fresh, preservatives must be added, many of which are harmful to our system. Such chemicals were believed to be safe in the past, but are not accepted as safe today. Those accepted today may be found to be harmful in the future. In the meantime, we continue to accumulate chemicals in our system and the effects may be noticed immediately, or over a longer period of time, or may even be transferred to the next generation.

Small farmers and producers who try to keep our food natural and wholesome cannot survive in competition with larger industries. Attempts have been made to synthesize natural food products and their vitamin and mineral content, but the nutritional efficiency of these synthetic products cannot be guaranteed. Many foods are bleached, colored, cured, dried, emulsified, enriched, flavored, preserved, refined, stabilized, sweetened, tenderized, or thickened. Such foods are devoid of their original, natural richness and should be avoided whenever possible. Let us look at some commonly used food products:

Fruits: Fruits are found in abundance and are generally inexpensive for the average person. They are light and easy to digest as well as satisfying to the appetite. Fruit is an excellent cleanser for the body and fruit fasting is highly recommended. The natural sweetness of fruit makes it an ideal dessert and is better than pastries, ice-cream, or candy. Fruits are divided into two categories, fresh and dried.

Fresh Fruits: Fresh fruits are either acid or sub-acid. Acid fruits are mainly citrus which are high in vitamin C and particularly cleansing for the body. Lemon juice, for example, taken daily improves elimination and relieves constipation problems. Limes, lemons, oranges, tangerines, grapefruit, berries, and pineapples are included in this category. Sub-acid fruits are sweet and their acid content is low. Bananas, avocados, grapes, peaches, plums, apples, etc. are in this category. Sub-acid fruits may be combined with other protein and acid foods.

Dried Fruits: Unlike fresh fruits, they are available during all seasons and can be easily stored. It is important to select those which are prepared without preservatives or sulphur. Many sweet dried fruits can be used with cereals and nuts, and are marvelous as snacks in place of cookies or candies. Prunes (a natural laxative), raisins (high in iron), dates, figs, and apricots are some of the fruits in this category.

Yoga highly recommends a fruit diet. It is the most Satvik, or pure type of food, and should be the main portion of the diet during the higher practices of Yoga.

Vegetables: Vegetables are the main source of vitamins and minerals needed by the body. They should be eaten raw as often as possible. If cooked, they should be steamed for a short time in order to preserve their vitamins and life force. Cover the pan while cooking and save the water they were steamed in as it is rich in food value. Use fresh vegetables whenever possible. If these are not available, use frozen rather than canned vegetables. Wash the skins as vegetables are often coated with wax or oil.

Fruit Bearing Vegetables: These grow above ground and have seeds. They are high in minerals and may be eaten raw, either alone or in combination, as in salads. Cucumbers, tomatoes, okra, and peppers are among these vegetables.

Root and Bulb Vegetables: These grow underground and are the roots of the plant. Many of them are excellent in salads. Garlic, horseradish, carrots, onions, beets, radishes, potatoes (white and sweet) are common examples. Most of these may be eaten raw, but it is best to bake the potatoes. The skins should always be eaten as they are high in potassium.

Green Vegetables are high in important vitamins and minerals, and many are natural laxatives. Spinach, celery, lettuce, string beans, and broccoli are among the green vegetables.

Juices: Juices are the simplest kind of food. They are easy to prepare, quick to digest, and are high in nutritional value. They contain important enzymes which are necessary for digestion of minerals. In addition they require less digestive energy than the fruits or vegetables from which the juice is made, and need only ten to fifteen minutes to be absorbed. Raw vegetable juices contain many organic elements which the body can utilize easily. Also, they have powerful building and regenerative value and are excellent when used as cures. They should be used immediately after preparation as many of their enzymes are destroyed in storage. Hydraulic juicers are believed to be the best because they masticate the fibers and the pulp, extracting the most important elements from them. Do not mix fruit and vegetable juices.

Milk and Dairy Products: Milk is a perfect food when it is consumed straight from the cow. In its original raw state, milk is high in protein, fats, calcium, and vitamins. Pasteurization destroys vitamin C, B-complex, and the enzymes needed to absorb calcium and phosphorous. Homogenization removes the cream and the flavor.

Cow's milk is mucus forming and should be avoided by people suffering from respiratory disorders and certain allergies. It may be replaced by goat's milk which is easier to digest. Low fat milk is desirable for people concerned about their weight.

Many milk products such as yogurt, buttermilk, sour cream, cheese, butter, cream cheese, and ice cream are high in protein, while products such as cottage cheese, ricotta cheese, and farmer's cheese are low in calories and are excellent combined with fresh fruits. Yogurt and buttermilk are high in lactic acid which is very useful in digestion and cleansing. They contain the friendly intestinal bacteria which are valuable to the stomach and intestines. The calcium in buttermilk and the protein contained in yogurt are gentler and easier to digest than that of regular milk. Yogurt is a natural antacid and should be eaten by those suffering from gas problems.

Nuts: Nuts are complete proteins. They should be eaten as snacks, preferably in their raw unsalted form. As nuts are high in fat and hard to digest, only a few should be eaten at a time. They should be chewed very well and, if possible, eaten early in the day. Children especially should be watched in this regard, as they may wind up with stomach pain and indigestion if they are not careful. Almonds, walnuts, peanuts, cashews, pecans, and pistachios are commonly available nuts.

Seeds: Sunflower seeds are 25% protein and a good source of vitamins and minerals. They have unsaturated fatty acid (vitamin F) which is high in calcium and methionine (an amino acid). The methionine content of sunflower seeds is greater than an equal amount of liver.

Sesame seeds are excellent in cakes and cookies. Their composition is similar to that of almonds and they are high in amino acids. Sesame oil is the most popular and commonly used oil in India. It has a unique and attractive flavor.

Legumes: Legumes include many dried beans such as lima, kidney, blackeye peas, peas, soy, and lentils. Soy beans can be prepared in a variety of ways. They are called the poor man's steak. The soy bean is an alkaline protein food, and does not need to be combined with anything else to maintain the alkaline-acid balance in the blood stream.

Grains and Cereals: Whole grains are high in protein, vitamins, and minerals. Stone ground wheat flour is particularly high in food value and should be used for baking if possible, in place of bleached white flour. Wheat germ is high in food value and may be included in bread, cereal, and many other preparations.

Yeast: Brewer's yeast is a good protein food. It is an excellent source of vitamin B-12, an essential vitamin for vegetarians. Yeast can be taken alone or combined with tomato juice, salads, or yogurt to improve the taste.

Bread: Bread is considered the staff of life. There are many bread companies which advertise the vitamin and mineral content of their breads, but they fail to mention the vital ingredients that are removed or the chemicals that are added. Most people are impressed by the advertisements and are satisfied with the taste so they never inquire further about its nutritional value.

Commercial bread contains many chemicals like methyl bromide, chlorine dioxide, and sodium propionate which are used to prolong shelf life and which may be harmful to our health.

The wheat kernel is composed of three major parts: Endosperm, bran, and germ. The endosperm comprises

83% of the kernel and is the major ingredient in white flour. It is made up largely of starch and cellulose. Bran comprises 14.5% of the kernel and is included in whole wheat flour but is not included in white flour. The germ comprises the remaining 2.5% of the wheat kernel. It is the embryo of the sprouting portion of the seed. As it contains fat which spoils flour in storage, it is removed from commercial white flour. Brans and the germs are the most nutritious portions of wheat; they are fed to farm animals and the starchy portion is left in white bread for human consumption. Chapter 24 includes recipes for wholesome breads containing whole wheat flour. Natural breads are available in health food stores in a variety of forms: yeast free, wheat free, multigrain, low sodium, and with dried fruit and nuts.

Salt or Sodium: Salt is a mineral which helps stabilize the acid-base balance in the body. It helps utilize carbohydrates and converts them into fat. Salt helps regulate the amount of water in the body cells. Excess salt, however, causes fluid retention which can result in hypertension due to lack of cell elasticity. Insufficient salt can cause fatigue, cramps, and retarded growth. Enough natural salt is found in raw fruits and vegetables so that little additional salt is necessary in cooking and eating. Use vege-salt made from raw dehydrated vegetables instead of commercial salt. Salt free diets are recommended for people with poor health and also in cases of certain ailments.

Sugar: Natural sugars like honey and molasses are recommended for daily consumption. Natural sugars contain thiamine (vitamin B-1) which helps the body metabolize the sugar. Molasses is a good source of iron and supplies extra oxygen to the blood stream, purifying the blood. Honey is absorbed quickly and easily and is rich in vitamins, minerals, and enzymes. Rapid absorption of the sugar in honey prevents fermentation as well as producing and sustaining body energy. It is also a good cleanser and a natural laxative. So many natural foods contain sufficient sugar that there is usually no need for additional refined sugar in our diet.

White, refined sugar is prepared commercially and contains no vitamins or minerals. It is a habit forming stimulant and does not help build the body. Instead, it adds empty calories which contribute to obesity, tooth decay, and hyperactivity. Commercial jams, jellies, candy, soft drinks, frostings, etc., contain refined sugar.

White sugar gives quick energy, but because certain important elements are removed, it is difficult to digest and overworks the internal organs. When sugar is consumed, the blood-sugar level increases and the pancreas secretes more insulin. This increase produces a temporary burst of energy, but soon the level drops to below normal and one may feel more fatigued than usual. White sugar destroys vitamin B-complex and disturbs the calcium-phosphorous balance, thus increasing the incidence of tooth decay.

Rice: Brown rice is high in protein and contains all of the important vitamins in proper proportion. It contains 37.5 grams of protein per pound. The refining process removes the complex vitamins as well as important protein and minerals; therefore, it is best to avoid white rice and minute rice altogether. Rice is mainly a carbohydrate food, and in its natural form is very wholesome. Orientals live on rice as their main food since it is not refined. Rice when combined with beans makes a complete protein.

Oils: Vegetable oil is preferable to animal oil as it is higher in unsaturated fat. Soya oil is a good source of protein and is frequently used in the recipes in this book. Use unrefined cold pressed or mechanically pressed oils.

Natural Laxative Foods: Use some of the following natural laxative foods in your diet as they have a natural cleansing effect.

Fruits: Figs, dates, apricots, prunes, peaches, pears, apples, grapes, oranges, grapefruits, and cantaloupes.

Raw Vegetables: Celery, radishes, cabbage, carrots, cucumbers, lettuce, tomatoes.

Cooked Vegetables: Beets, turnips, lentils, cauliflower, spinach, string beans, whole grain cereals.

Beverages: Use herb teas as beverages instead of soda, alcoholic drinks, tea, or coffee. Herb teas have a very pleasant flavor as well as a cleansing effect on the body. Most health food stores have a variety of herb teas. Milk is a food so don't use it as a beverage. Drink water frequently during the day since it is the best body cleanser. Juices of fresh fruits and vegetables are very healthy beverages.

HOLISTIC HEALTH PRODUCTS

There is a growing interest in the vegetarian diet, health foods, and holistic health approaches. As the public becomes more aware and concerned about their health, manufacturers are becoming involved and producing varieties of natural foods. Following are examples of this trend:

1. Herbs and herbal combinations for natural remedies.

2. Homeopathic preparations are composed of small concentrations of nutrients to help the body heal itself.

3. Ayurvedic preparations are for nutrition and health care.

4. Aloe Vera has been developed in tonic and cosmetic forms.

5. Natural energy products such as bee pollen, ginseng, herbal compositions, stress vitamins, chlorophyll, spirulina, barley grass, wheat grass.

6. Body building products which include protein drinks, glandulars, antioxidants, and antiaging nutrition.

7. Internal cleansing compounds: complete programs for colon health; i.e., psyllium husks, bran, fibers, etc.

8. Free form amino acids developed for weight control and neuronutrition.

9. Specialized products: yeast, salt, sugar, and wheat free. Low cholesterol, low calories, unprocessed foods.

10. Vegetarian substitutes for burgers, hot dogs, steaks, meat balls, bacon, etc. made from vegetarian protein in frozen, canned (lead free) and bulk form, ready-cooked or easy to cook forms available.

MACROBIOTICS

Macrobiotic is an ancient concept of Hindu, Chinese, Japanese, and Hebrew cultures. Macrobiotic means prolonging life by a balanced diet and a balanced life style. Originally it was introduced 160 years ago by Christopher Hufeland, a German research professor. Dr. Oshawa elaborated on this concept and established his dietary system using the traditional Japanese diet, and it became known in the West as the macrobiotic diet. This diet should be modified to use locally available products.

Macrobiotic principles are:
1. Eat locally grown food and in season
2. Eat whole and uncontaminated food.
3. Maintain an acid-alkaline balance of diet within the Yin and Yang principles.

Macrobiotic diet uses the following guidelines for producing Yin and Yang balance:
1. 50-60% whole grains
2. 5% each of soup, sea vegetables, condiments
3. 20-25% cooked vegetables 5% raw vegetables
4. 5-10% beans

A macrobiotic diet excludes dairy products which make it a mucusless diet and has been proven to be effective against cancer, colds, and other diseases. The absence of mucus retards the growth of organisms and speeds up the healing process.

Although the macrobiotic diet provides balanced nutrition, one should remain flexible and make adjustments to suit one's constitution, climate, and activities. One should follow this diet strictly in case of a special physical need and under the guidance of an expert. This diet should be introduced gradually into the system, as sudden restrictions of certain nutritious foods and elimination of all dairy products will produce physical and mental stress. This will, in turn, push one to indulgence and rebellion against the basic principles of macrobiotics causing further stress and guilt.

TAO - Balance of Yin and Yang

The concept of an absolute, eternal, and infinite universe was known to ancient China over 5000 years ago. This infinite universe differentiated itself into Yin and Yang principles which began the process of physical and material manifestation of our relative world.

Around 600 B.C. Confucius wrote I Ching and Lao Tzu wrote Tao Teh Ching which elaborate the principles of Yin and Yang which can be applied at the individual and social levels, and which have influenced the way of life in Eastern countries.

Yin and Yang are the two arms of infinity within which everything is constantly changing. Everything begins and ends, ultimately balancing out. Opposing forces like pleasure and pain, day and night, love and hate, male and female, etc. complement each other.

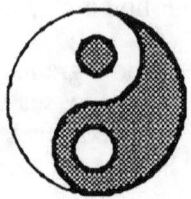

This principle is similar to the Samkhya philosophy of Yoga where the Impersonal God, Brahman, is expressed by the male aspect Krishna, Shiva, or consciousness; and the female aspect is expressed by Radha, Shakti, or universal energy. This universal energy fluctuates constantly with the three forces of nature: Satva, Rajas, and Tamas, and these forms manifest as our material universe.

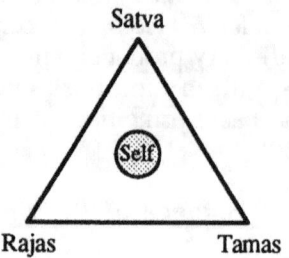

When these forces attain equilibrium, the physical universe returns to its undifferentiated, unmanifest form.

The principles of Tao and Samkhya Yoga agree on the fact that the universe is in a constant state of flux. We cannot control it, make it all good, or remove evil from it. We can only learn to tune into the rhythm of the universe and learn to flow with it, finding harmony and peace.

Ultimately one can transcend nature and experience the higher reality (Brahman).

YIN AND YANG FOODS

The foods we eat also contain Yin and Yang properties. Some foods are mildly Yin or Yang while others are strongly Yin or Yang. These qualities are relative and one should choose the proper combination of foods to establish a delicate balance between the two.

Yin food: These foods grow in hot climates and are juicy, soft, big, and cook quickly. They include tropical fruits, vegetables, and alcohol. They are cooling and slow you down.

Yang food: These foods grow in colder climates and are dry, small, hard, and require longer cooking time. Examples include beans, nuts, meat, salt, fish, and eggs. Yang foods warm the body and stimulate energy.

Saturate your mind and feelings with abundance. This will allow you to rise above restless desires. When you feel saturated you feel contentment.

If you pray to the Lord He will provide whatever you want, which may or may not satisfy you. If you ask for nothing but Divine Love, wisdom, and guidance he will fulfill all your needs and will make you free.

Keep away from bad company/association. Their negative influence will rub off on you no matter how careful you are. Going into a coal mine you cannot avoid getting dirty by the soot of the charcoal.

Natural and Health Foods

21

VEGETARIANISM

When a student of Yoga reads about vegetarianism the first question he asks is why should anyone become a vegetarian? The question I would ask is why should anyone eat meat? The vegetarian diet is natural for humans who were originally vegetarian until they were pushed into meat eating due to lack of food.

Nature has manufactured different biological structures and body chemistry for herbivorous and carnivorous animals. Humans, cows, horses, elephants, etc. are herbivorous while cats, dogs, lions, etc. are carnivorous.

All meat eating animals have sharp front teeth and claws to tear the meat. They also have smaller salivary glands which secrete acidic saliva. Vegetarian animals and humans have flat back molar teeth to grind food and well developed salivary glands that secrete alkaline saliva to predigest the carbohydrates in grains.

Meat eating animals have strong hydrochloric acid in their stomaches to digest tough meat while vegetarian animals secrete relatively mild hydrochloric acid for digesting vegetarian protein. Carnivorous animals have shorter intestinal tracts so meat is digested and waste eliminated quickly. Herbivorous animals have longer intestinal tracts which allow absorption of a variety of nutrients over a longer period of time.

Animals instinctively choose the correct diet; humans don't follow natural laws.

Nonviolence is the most important discipline in Yoga. One must have compassion for all living creatures. In the Christian commandments it is said, "Thou shall not kill." If we cannot produce life we have no right to destroy it. Yoga philosophy advocates reincarnation with the law of cause and effect. All causes have their effects and eventually we must pay for killing animals and causing their suffering. When people eat meat they see only the steak and not the live animal behind it. If one could visualize the animal he just might not be able to eat meat.

A sure way to realize the violence and suffering involved in meat eating is to visit a slaughterhouse. Seeing the suffering of the animals would make us think twice before eating their flesh. A Hindu who has never thought of meat eating would get sick at the thought of eating it, just as a meat eater might get sick at the thought of eating worms, ants, or snakes. After becoming used to something one does not think about it and becomes insensitive to it. People who are introduced to meat eating from childhood, eat meat out of habit. With the practice of Yoga one becomes more sensitive to feelings and vibrations, especially of living beings, and then their love expands to all life. Advanced Yogis can expand their love so powerfully that even wild creatures of the jungle become pets in their presence; criminals become as saints, and disturbed people find peace of mind. Animals have especially strong instincts and in holy places of pilgrimage in India where people feed and respect them, they become friendly.

Many spiritually advanced persons in the past have been vegetarians, for when one practices Yoga, the body becomes purified, meat and junk food are rejected, and natural food is desired. Many practitioners have the desire to give up meat but they do not know what to eat instead. A vegetarian diet is not made up of vegetables alone; it includes a variety of foods with satisfying taste and more than sufficient nourishment. Included are fresh fruits, vegetables, nuts, beans, dairy products, and a variety of grains. It excludes all meat, fish, sea food, and other foods containing animal life. Some strict vegetarians exclude milk and dairy products. Yogis recommend cow's milk and many of them remain on a milk diet for months during the sadhana (spiritual practices). In India milk is a wholesome food because it is neither pasteurized nor homogenized. Cows are worshiped and respected as mothers and their milk is accepted as mothers' milk. Excess milk is taken from the cow only after her calf is properly fed. This process involves no violence.

The dairy industry in the United States feeds the cow a great deal of nutritious food in a short period of time in order to speed up the milk producing process. This milk is lacking in some important nutrients and the poor cow becomes run-down. Milk is taken from the cow by mechanical monsters with no consideration given to the calves. The prison atmosphere seems to become routine for the cow who will be sent to the slaughterhouse when her milk production ceases to be profitable.

It is an individual decision whether or not to include dairy products in the diet. Eggs are not permitted in the vegetarian diet, but some people eat them if they are not fertilized. According to Yoga our body is only an outer shell and we must rise above it. Eating meat makes you more attached to the gross physical body by increasing the lower passions. When we are attached to our physical body we become a slave to it. We have to rise above the body to the level of mind and intellect, ultimately coming to the level of consciousness. By eating a pure vegetarian diet we increase our ability to concentrate, meditate, and eventually become our true nature which is pure consciousness.

A vegetarian diet is perfect for humans. Vegetables derive their energy from the earth, water, and sunshine. They are high in vitamins and minerals and, as they are a primary form of food, they are easily consumed and assimilated by the body. Much of vegetarian food can be sprouted as it is alive and absorbs atmospheric energy. Also, it breaks down easily providing quick energy without taxing the digestive organs.

Meat is a secondary form of food and takes longer to digest, therefore it requires the use of more vital energy. The net gain of energy in vegetarianism is greater than that gained from a meat diet. Meat produces stiffness of joints and muscles, and lethargy, while a vegetarian diet keeps the body supple which is conducive to the practice of Yoga positions and yogic breathing techniques. Meat has been converted from plant life and the molecules are complex and difficult for our system to digest. Although it is high in protein, it is low in many vitamins and minerals and contains large amounts of uric acid and saturated fats which are the cause of many health problems.

The metabolism of excess protein leaves a toxic residue in body tissues causing auto toxemia (overacidity) and nutritional deficiency. Meat contains a greater ratio of phosphorous to calcium and this can cause a calcium deficiency. As excess uric acid accumulates and is deposited in various organs, diseases such as gout, rheumatism, headaches, and nervousness result. Saturated fat, which is high in lower grades of meat, causes problems such as hardening of the arteries and high blood pressure which are unknown to vegetarians. An extra intake of uric acid must be eliminated by the body and this increases the work load for the liver and kidneys.

Many pesticides are used in growing vegetarian foods. Vegetables themselves have a low concentration of them, but when animals eat pesticides their fat tissues retain them (such as DDT) and the concentration increases. Meat eating, therefore, increases pesticide consumption and retention in the human body.

Animal protein putrefies twice as fast as vegetable protein and many diseases are produced by protein putrefaction in the intestines. The human intestinal passage is very long which allows meat to decay and may cause colon cancer. Meat protein is more toxic when combined with other foods as compared with vegetable protein. Also, due to tension and fear at the time of slaughter, animals release a highly toxic secretion of adrenaline which is carried into their meat causing anxiety to the consumer. In accordance with today's meat producing practices animals are raised on a large scale under unnatural conditions. They are force-fed and fattened in a short time rather than being allowed the normal period for growth, causing inferior meat. This fattening process produces external fat which is then removed as a waste product. A slow and natural process of feeding produces a higher quality meat, but it is not economical.

Animals are capable of digesting humanly inedible food and of converting it into protein. Today, however, they are fed valuable and humanly edible foods because it is less expensive. Many pounds of protein are fed to animals to produce one pound of meat. If this vegetarian protein were fed to people directly, it would fill many more stomachs. Also, animal parasites are easily transferred to humans when they eat meat.

A common argument against vegetarianism is that meat is high in protein and what can you substitute for it? Beans and nuts are good sources of protein and much more economical than meat. Soya beans have been called the poor man's steak for they contain about three times as much protein as an equal amount of boneless meat.

Recent research indicates that we need only 25 to 30 grams of protein a day to maintain ideal health. In vegetarian countries where people enjoy good health and longevity, they consume very small amounts of protein and a great amount of complex carbohydrates. The average American eats more protein than necessary, and this excess protein is converted into carbohydrates providing extra calories and weight gain.

Vegetarians have longer lasting energy and more endurance. Meat eaters have bigger and stronger muscles but become exhausted in a short time; they also lack the mental sharpness and serenity of vegetarians. According to Yoga, a meat eater's energy is Rajasik, a lower form of energy which brings restlessness, tension, and fear. If this energy is not properly channeled it could be self-destructive. Energy gained by eating a properly balanced vegetarian diet brings Satvik energy which produces purity of body, balanced emotions, and a calm mind.

NONVIOLENCE

As we evolve spiritually, compassion for all living creatures increases. One doesn't desire to kill animals for pleasure. Instead man, being superior in intelligence, becomes responsible for protecting animals.

When there is plenty of vegetarian food available we cannot think of eating animals for survival. In the history of mankind man chose to eat them only when there was need due to a shortage of food, climate conditions, or other geographical situations.

There is no limit as to how far one can progress in a vegetarian diet. One may become a vegan, giving up dairy products and honey, or become a fruitarian. The diet should be chosen according to one's personal evolution. We can never remain completely nonviolent as plants have life too and we kill germs simply by breathing. Yoga scriptures teach that one life lives on another life. This is the law of nature which has created the cycle of evolution. Within our own body the cells are killing each other all the time.

Purity of diet is used only as a means to purify our consciousness in order to realize that I am Brahman. My consciousness is a reflection of Brahman while the body is part of the universal nature (Prakriti).

In time, one transcends the superficial moral code of nonviolence and sees God in all living things. A prayer before eating, as mentioned in the Gita, states: "This food is Brahman, the fire of the stomach is Brahman, the process of eating is Brahman. Brahman goes to Brahman. Everything is homogeneous in Brahman." By reciting this prayer aloud or mentally, one purifies the food and accepts it as Prasad (blessings of God). In this way, one purifies his consciousness. One should utilize this human birth for Self-realization and should not become preoccupied with food. As we realize that what comes out of our mouth is more important than what goes in, we should express our sweetness through thoughts, words, and deeds. It is useless to be a strict vegetarian while offending the world by thoughts, words, or deeds.

CAUTION: Those who are meat eaters should not change to a vegetarian diet suddenly as this could be a shock to the system. Slowly reduce the intake of meat while increasing the vegetarian diet. Some people use fish and sea food as a transition diet before changing to pure vegetarianism. Health food stores contain many new products which provide a meat substitute similar in taste, texture, and protein. These stores have a good supply of frozen, packaged, and canned foods as well as a variety of vegetarian cookbooks

There should be no conflict between material and spiritual life. Reality is where our heart is. If our heart is on God, all our material activities are spiritualized. If our heart is in the world, our spiritual activities become worldly activities.

A jar may be full but when shaken, the contents may settle down and make room for more. By shaking and adjusting our priorities, we can find time for worthwhile things in life.

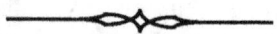

Satsang provides spiritual energy. In the forest fire green trees burn up easily along with the dry trees. A person finds spiritual strength in group satsang.

Be like a python. He accepts his prey as it comes to him instead of running after it. Be content with whatever comes to you naturally instead of hankering after any attainments.

22

FASTING

In Sanskrit the word for fasting is Oopvas. Oop means closer and vas means living. It is an art of staying closer to God. Most religions of the world recommend some kind of fasting and many advocate abstinence from certain foods. Hindus and Yogis fast for physical and mental purification and for spiritual communion with God. While fasting is well known in India, in the West there has always been a fear of dying of starvation due to fasting. Recent experiments have shown that fasting with proper knowledge cannot kill anyone. In fact, more people die of overeating than of starvation. Overeating, even of the most nourishing foods, can cause disease and malnutrition. An important lesson can be learned from animals who instinctively obey the laws of nature, eating only when they are hungry and fasting when they are sick. Humans, on the other hand, eat primarily to satisfy the palate.

Any machine that works must rest, or it will overheat and break down. People who work need a week-end to rest if they expect to maintain efficiency. Likewise, our body and mind need one day a week for a rest period. This rest produces rejuvenation not only for all the vital internal organs but also for the mind. Overworked organs of the body do not function efficiently and subsequently their life span is reduced. Digestion and elimination involve many organs including the heart, liver, and kidneys. Fasting provides a much needed rest for these organs and, at the same time, one's energy is redirected toward cleansing and purifying the body of toxins.

During a fast, the pores of the skin eliminate toxic wastes. The lungs eliminate poisons which can be noticed in the form of bad breath; the tongue gets a white, toxic coating indicating the cleansing process, and urine is darker due to toxic elimination. Improper elimination of waste is a major cause of bodily disorders. Morbid waste from the organs and tissues congest the blood stream causing disease. As these impurities are removed during fasting, the blood becomes purified. When the body is free of toxins, nature can perform its healing and sustaining work.

An English translation of fasting implies fastening or holding with a purpose. We fast with a definite purpose in mind. A proper mental attitude must be assumed and maintained, otherwise, fasting becomes starving. There are short and long term fasts. The short term may last from one to three days and is safe to perform without supervision providing there are no specific prohibitive physical reasons not to fast. Short term fasting is used primarily for cleansing. A longer fast may range from four days to a month or more and is useful for a thorough cleansing and for curing certain diseases. It should be done under the guidance of an experienced naturopathic practitioner. Short fasts may be carried on during normal activities; longer fasts require bed rest.

Long Term Fast: Long fasts are recommended during the deeper practices of Yoga and for curing chronic diseases. The most effective long term fast is a pure water fast. After the first three days of a water fast the body will begin burning its own tissues, starting with old damaged tissues and wastes stored in the body. This also speeds up the building of new cells. A water fast generates physical weakness and requires bed rest. The healing benefits come when the fast is broken.

Long fasts remove the strong hold of the lower passions, and one can easily feel communion with God. Long fasting is a great spiritual discipline, and it is recommended that all serious Yoga practitioners do a seven to ten day fast at least once a year. Read a detailed book on this subject to receive thorough guidance before you begin. Also prepare your mind psychologically.

Breaking the fast is more critical than the fast itself. One should break the fast very gradually to avoid a burden to the stomach. After three or four days of fasting hunger leaves, and within four to ten days the weakness leaves. One feels stronger than before fasting. This increased strength is evidence that a person who feels sluggish and tired may not be lacking in nutrition, but rather his condition may be due to toxins in the body. If these toxins are released from the body too quickly one becomes sick and may be advised to stop the fast. Real hunger returns from the 21st to the 60th day depending upon the individual. One must stop fasting at this time as starvation and health damage begin beyond this point.

Juice Fast: It is safer and more enjoyable to fast using raw juices and vegetable broths. (Do not mix vegetable and fruit juices.) These juices provide vitamins, minerals, and enzymes without taxing the digestive organs. They also provide an alkaline surplus which neutralizes acid waste and provides a general mineral balance in the cells. Juice fasting promotes quick regeneration of new cells as old ones are destroyed. This provides a pleasant healthy fast without feeling the hunger pain or weakness of a water fast.

Short Term Fast: Yoga recommends moderation in diet, eating less, eating nutritious health foods, and fasting regularly once a week for twenty-four hours. If you maintain the rhythm of fasting on the same day of the week your body will become adjusted to it. Begin with a partial or fruit and juice fast until you can fast on water alone. Fast through breakfast, lunch, and dinner continuing daily work but avoiding heavy labor. Fasting removes natural thirst so be sure to drink plenty of water, at least five glasses a day. Water should be at room temperature and sipped slowly. It is a good cleanser, diluting the urine and cleansing the kidneys. Break the fast the following morning by drinking fresh fruit or vegetable juice at room temperature. It may also be broken with a light salad. Avoid a heavy lunch, but eat a normal dinner. If you find it difficult to follow these fasting times, begin fasting from lunch and break it with a light lunch the next day.

A lukewarm water enema once a month on the evening of the fast day is recommended. After the enema drink some warm herbal tea or room temperature juice. This will prevent reabsorption of the waste loosened by the enema.

SUGGESTIONS AND RULES FOR FASTING

If you are not used to fasting, begin gently. First, omit only one meal at a time, gradually increasing fasting periods as your system becomes accustomed to it. Partial fasts can be carried on by people who cannot fast on water. They may drink one kind or a variety of fruit juices during the fast. Partial benefits are obtained by fruit and juice fasts.

It is not a valid fast if you do not eat because you are not hungry. The real cleansing takes place during the time you feel very hungry. If you don't feel hungry due to ill health you are not fasting. Without proper mental preparation fasting becomes starving.

Fast on the same day each week as this assures regular rest for the stomach and entire body. Choose your fasting day when physical activities are light, but you will be mentally busy. Also, do not take vitamins during your fast as they should interact with food to provide nourishment and are wasted if taken alone. Your body has an adequate reserve to support you during the fast.

Some beginners experience weakness, dizziness, headaches, and other problems during fasting. The sensation of hunger is a nerve impulse due to a lifetime eating habit. It is not true hunger. Persons fasting for a long time report that this impulse dies away. Drinking citrus juices will alleviate this problem as well as provide a cleansing effect and supply quick energy without overburdening the digestive system. You may do yogic deep breathing to charge your body with prana instead of drinking juices.

Sometimes physical discomforts during fasts are created by toxins which are being eliminated. If you have any temptation to break the fast, renew your will power by remembering the benefits or read a book on fasting.

Many factors must be considered when fasting: age, physical condition, weight, and the nature of work performed during the fast. People with low blood sugar, diabetics, young children, and underweight people must be particularly careful and should do partial rather than complete fasting.

Never break the fast with a heavy meal as this will create a burden for the stomach. When fasting more than one day, eat only salads or simple foods the day before and the day after the fast. An occasional enema at night is necessary for longer fasts. There are also colon cleansing products on the market which are especially beneficial during a fast.

The day following the fast you will experience lightness and rejuvenation of the body. You will wake up feeling refreshed, with a good appetite, and the simple foods you did not care for before will be new and interesting to you. Tension and laziness will be gone, and the body will become flexible. Yoga postures will be performed with ease, and breathing control will improve.

In Yoga practice, fasting is the first step towards purification. The mind is the finer substance of the body and is calmed and mellowed by fasting. While the body loses weight and strength the mind becomes sharp and one pointed, untroubled by distractions. Fasting is required before one is initiated into the higher states of Yoga training. According to Yoga, we have astral nerve tubes called nadis which correspond to the sensory and motor nerves. These nadis are purified by fasting and yogic breathing.

Fasting reduces passion and restlessness. One who disciplines the palate can discipline the sensual desires and can direct the sensual energy to spiritual growth. Also, while resting the body one becomes more and more aware of himself and has a chance to know himself in the true sense, becoming aware of the functions of the body and mind. Fasting converts animal man to spiritual man.

According to Yoga our life span is determined by the number of breaths taken per minute. Regularity of breath and the length of the breath determine our emotional state. Fasting makes the breathing rhythmic and slower which calms the nerves and extends our life span.

No man can serve two masters. There are two boats, one is going toward the world, the other is going toward God. You cannot keep one foot in each boat. You must choose one of them.

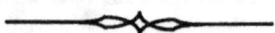

The sun gives light and warmth unconditionally. A tree gives fruits to friends and foes alike. One should learn to give unconditionally.

Desires are more poisonous than a cobra. A cobra kills only once, but desires kill you many times.

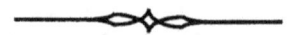

23

CLEANSING

In addition to fasting, there are other simple cleansing techniques recommended in Yoga. Our body eliminates toxins through the following organs: the tongue, nostrils, eyes, bladder, colon, skin, and lungs. Many vital organs such as the stomach, kidneys, liver, and digestive organs are also involved in removing waste. The kidneys maintain water balance and eliminate waste through the urinary tract. The liver filters the blood and restores nutrients, sending its waste into the colon. Following are descriptions of recommended cleansing techniques:

METHODS OF CLEANSING

1. Drink Plenty of Water

In the morning upon rising drink a large glass of warm water. You may squeeze some lemon juice into it. During the night waste in the colon dries out as in the last stage of digestion most of the moisture is absorbed by the large intestine. This practice will eliminate constipation problems. Water, unlike tea and coffee (which are habit forming stimulants), is the most natural cleansing beverage. Excess water will also help flush the kidneys.

Throughout the day one should drink about five glasses of water, sipped slowly at room temperature. Cold water is hard on the digestive system. Don't drink water during or immediately after meals as this dilutes the digestive juices. Many modern city and well water systems are contaminated. Use a good reliable filter to remove harmful contaminants.

Spring water is ideal for everyday use as it provides important minerals for the body. Make sure it is not contaminated. Distilled water contains no minerals and is ideal to use during fasting, but regular use of distilled water will extract essential minerals from your body. If using distilled water, take a chelated or orotate mineral supplement daily.

2. Eyes

Clean your eyes with distilled water. If this is not available, boil water and then allow it to cool. Open the eyes wide and sprinkle them with the water, then open and shut them several times. This improves eyesight as well as cleanses. Do this every day preferably in the morning, and it will help you feel refreshed and wide awake.

3. Tongue

Brush your teeth every morning upon rising, then clean your tongue. During the night toxins are deposited on the tongue in the form of a white coating. This can be removed with a tongue cleaner, preferably made of stainless steel. It may be available at health food stores. The tongue scraper is about 8" long and 1/4" wide, reasonably sharp, and is shaped into a U form. The rounded part is placed in the mouth while the tongue is pulled out and the white coating is scraped off. The tongue indicates the stomach's condition. Therefore, more of a white coating indicates an unhealthy stomach condition. During fasting more toxins accumulate on the tongue due to the cleansing process. Cleaning the tongue in this manner produces a refreshing feeling, reduces mouth odors, gum disease, plaque, and is hygienic. Once you use this method, you will never skip it. It is much better than using a toothbrush as the bristles damage taste buds, and it is not as sanitary a method.

4. Lungs

Cleansing breathing purifies the lungs as explained in Chapter 6, Breathing. The Lion position removes stale, congested air by squeezing the lungs and is explained in Chapter 5, Yoga Positions.

5. Nasal Passages

Clean the nostrils and sinus passages everyday. Add 1/4 teaspoon of salt to a glass of warm water, making a saline solution. Place some of this solution in the palm of your hand and gently sniff the solution. Inhale the water and blow it out through the nostrils until you can inhale the water comfortably, forcing it out through the mouth. When the nasal passage is cleaned, there is no harm if a little water is swallowed. It is not as difficult as it may seem. Once you are used to it you can clean the entire passage in one or two minutes. This clears nasal congestion and makes breathing easier. It is especially helpful if you have a cold.

6. Skin

The skin is the largest eliminative organ, releasing about one pound of waste a day. Thus, it is called the third kidney. The pores of the skin are also involved with breathing, providing oxygen and eliminating carbon dioxide. It absorbs many nutrients by exposure to sunshine or contact with the ocean. Allow the skin to breathe by wearing nonsynthetic clothing and use only natural cosmetics.

Your skin can be stimulated and cleansed after bathing by rubbing it with a rough bath towel until it becomes red. A much better method is a dry brush massage. By using a vegetable fiber massage brush, the entire surface of the body should be brushed (except the face) beginning with the feet using circular motions. This should be done before showering on a daily basis, but is particularly beneficial during a fast. Dry brush massage removes dead layers of skin, metabolic wastes and impurities, and removes many toxins from the body. It stimulates the blood capillaries and nerve endings, and unclogs the lymphatic system. Sweat glands are opened and cellulite is reduced. As the skin throws out uric acid and other metabolic wastes, it removes the burden from the liver and kidneys. The natural beauty of the skin is revealed.

7. Colon

The colon is the sewer system of our body and when it gets clogged the entire body is affected in one way or another. To maintain optimum health the colon should be cleaned regularly.

Due to contamination in our food, impure water and air, and wrong diets and habits over a period of years, our colon becomes overloaded and clogged with black, dry, putrefied matter deposited on the inner lining. Small amounts of dehydrated feces adhere permanently to the intestinal walls. Consequently the opening becomes narrow and this results in poorly functioning valves on both sides of the colon. A poorly functioning colon allows the body to reabsorb toxic residue; the blood picks up these impurities and circulates them through the entire body, resulting in contamination. The burden of elimination is then transferred to the skin causing skin problems, bad breath, indigestion, and premature aging. Impurities are then deposited in the joints and muscles. Headaches, tension, and lethargy set in. A clogged colon promotes harmful bacteria which cause many problems.

A. Acidophilus: The colon contains both friendly and unfriendly bacteria. The friendly bacteria are necessary to form some B-vitamins and to fight harmful organisms. Use yogurt in your diet or take acidophilus capsules to insure a good supply of intestinal flora. Avoid antibiotics if at all possible as they kill the friendly bacteria. If you must take them, be sure and supplement with extra acidophilus.

B. Fasting and Enema: The colon is cleansed during a water or juice fast. At the end of the fast one should take a warm water enema to remove waste from the colon.

C. Yoga Positions: Many Yoga positions help with internal cleansing. For example, the abdominal lift and stomach churning are ideal for massaging internal organs and also help with colon cleansing.

D. Fibers: Fibers are those portions of fruits, vegetables, and grains that the body does not break down during digestion. Fibers can be soluble or insoluble, and they help with the elimination process. Soluble fiber is the gummy portion in fruits, beans, oatmeal, etc. It forms a gel that thickens food and slows down the digestive process and keeps you feeling full for a long period of time which helps prevent overeating. Glucomanon, Guar Gum, Guarana, etc. are fiber products used for suppressing hunger. Soluble fiber helps reduce blood cholesterol, gives prolonged energy, and binds and removes carcinogens (cancer causing agents).

Insoluble fiber is the crunchy part in bran, whole grains, and cereals. It holds moisture, provides roughage, increases peristaltic action, and helps force out waste from the colon. Shortening the transit time for waste removal reduces the chance for colon contamination.

One needs total fiber (soluble and insoluble) for optimum benefits. These fibers can be purchased from health food stores and should include fruit, vegetable, and grain fibers. Researchers recommend 20 to 35 gm. fiber per day. If you do not get this through your food, use the mixed fiber daily .

E. Internal Cleansing Programs: Health food stores carry a variety of intestinal cleansing programs. Some are quick and intensive while others are milder and take a longer time. Everyone should go through a thorough cleansing program two to four times a year along with a water or juice fast, or light diet. Such cleansing will remove old waste and rejuvenate the body and mind. Anyone with a chronic ailment will find tremendous relief after the cleansing program because all problems are rooted directly or indirectly in the colon. After the cleansing program it becomes easier to begin any new discipline such as a diet change, becoming vegetarian, quitting smoking, etc.

One may use psyllium husk powder or capsules along with acidophilus as a daily maintenance program. Psyllium husk is one of the major ingredients in these programs. In addition, a daily maintenance program will help provide necessary fiber, control the appetite, and maintain a healthy colon.

To be lazy and postpone things (procrastination) is basic human nature. Imagine that you have only one month to live, and you will be able to set priorities and act on important issues of life.

College education begins after graduating from high school. Spiritual life begins after graduating from material life. One has to fulfill and transcend material obligations and not use spiritual life as an escape from material responsibilities.

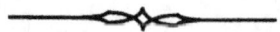

Forgive yourself and you will be able to forgive others. Love yourself and you will be able to love others.

24

VEGETARIAN RECIPES

SOUPS

Cooking beans using a pressure cooker

Do not put beans directly into the cooker because as the skins come lose they may clog the vent. First, place two cups of water into the cooker. Place the beans in a separate container with water and transfer them to the pressure cooker, then close the cooker and cook them. Different beans require different amounts of cooking time. For example, mung beans and lentils cook in 15 minutes while chick peas take 30 minutes.

Cooking beans without a pressure cooker

Soak the beans in water for about 3 hours. Chick peas, soya beans, green peas, etc. require longer soaking time (or overnight). Beans require more water for cooking when cooked without pressure cooker.

BEAN SOUPS

Aduki Bean

1 cup beans	1 tsp. salt
2 cups water	1/4 tsp. turmeric
1 Tbs. soya oil	1/2 tsp. curry powder
1/4 tsp. mustard seeds	1 tsp. coriander powder
3 cups water	2 tsp. grated coconut
1 cup stewed or	2 tsp. sugar
4 fresh chopped tomatoes	1 Tbs. fresh ground garlic

Cook beans in pressure cooker for 15 minutes. In another container heat the oil, add mustard seeds. After they pop, add beans and all ingredients. Mix well with a beater to break the beans to make thicker soup. Boil for 10 minutes.

Lentil, mung beans, mixed beans (limas, blackeye peas, and chick peas), green peas, and other beans can be cooked the same way. 5 to 6 servings.

Mung Bean Broth

1/2 cup mung beans
3 cups water
1 tsp. salt
1 tsp. ground or chopped fresh ginger

1 tsp. cumin powder
1 tsp. lemon juice
1 tsp. chopped coconut

Cook beans with water in pressure cooker for 10 minutes. Cool. In a separate container transfer the cooked beans. Add all ingredients. Mix with a beater and then boil for 5 minutes.

This soup is easy to digest and may be used to break a fast or during illness.

Spinach with Split Mung Beans (or Lentils)

1 cup split mung beans
(or lentils)
2 cups water
5 cups chopped fresh spinach (or 24 oz. frozen)
3 chopped onions
1/2 chopped green pepper
1 Tbs. oil

1/2 tsp. cumin seeds
2 tsp. salt
1/2 tsp. turmeric
1 tsp. coriander powder
2 Tbs. sesame seeds
2 Tbs. lemon juice
3 cups water

Cook beans in pressure cooker with 2 cups of water for 10 minutes. In another container heat oil and add cumin seeds. When they turn brown add spinach, the cooked beans, and the rest of the ingredients. Boil for 10 minutes. Add water as necessary to thin the soup.

VEGETABLE SOUPS

Fresh Tomato Soup

10 to 12 fresh chopped tomatoes

1 tsp. cumin seeds
1 tsp. ground black pepper

3 cups water   2 tsp. sugar
1 tsp. salt   grated cheese

Mix all ingredients except cheese and cook for 10 minutes. Cool
and blend in a blender. Strain to remove skin and seeds. Boil
and serve. Top with grated cheese. 5 to 6 servings.

Vegetable Broth

3 cups chopped fresh   1/4 tsp. ground black
vegetables (broccoli,   pepper
potatoes, carrots, celery,   1 tsp. parsley leaves
lettuce, etc.)   1/2 tsp. oregano leaves
2 cups water   3/4 cup yogurt
1 tsp. salt

Cook the vegetables and spices together in a pressure cooker for
5 minutes, or without pressure cooker add more water and cook
for 15 minutes. Cool. Blend in a blender with yogurt. Strain if
desired. Boil for 2 minutes. Serve. Add water to thin the soup
as necessary.
This broth is tasty and light. It is suitable to eat to break a weekly
one day fast. Serves 3.

Mixed Vegetable Soup

3 Tbs. oil   6 cups water
1 tsp. cumin seed   1 Tbs. salt
1 cup stewed tomatoes or   1 Tbs. parsley leaves
fresh chopped tomatoes   1 Tbs. oregano leaves
8 cups chopped fresh   1 Tbs. chopped garlic
vegetables   2 Tbs. sugar
(broccoli, cauliflower, carrots,
celery, string beans, cabbage, green peas)

In a large sauce-pan heat cumin seeds in oil until brown. Add
tomatoes and the rest of the ingredients. Cook at medium heat
for 20 minutes or until vegetables are cooked. Beat with a beater
if you desire to thicken the soup. Serve.

Barley Vegetable Soup

1 cup barley
2 cups water
1 Tbs. oil
1 tsp. cumin seeds
1 cup stewed (or 4 or 5 fresh) tomatoes
1/2 cup chopped string beans
1/2 cup chopped celery

1/2 cup chopped carrots
1 tsp. salt
1 Tbs. fresh chopped garlic
1 Tbs. oregano leaves
1 Tbs. parsley leaves
2 Tbs. coconut
3 cups water

Cook barley in pressure cooker for 15 minutes. In separate container heat oil, add cumin seeds. When they turn brown, add tomatoes and vegetables and cook for 5 minutes. Then add barley, remaining spices, and 3 cups of water. Boil for 10 minutes. 5 to 6 servings.

RICE

Plain Brown Rice I

1 cup rice   2 cups water

Place the rice in a container. Rinse once or twice with water. Add 2 cups of water and transfer it to the pressure cooker. Cook 15 minutes. 3 servings.

Plain Brown Rice II

1 Tbs. oil   1 cup rice   2 cups water

In a sauce-pan heat the oil and add rice. Stir constantly over low heat for 3 minutes or until light brown, then add water. Cover the pan and cook at high heat. When it begins to boil reduce the heat and cook at low heat for 30 minutes or until rice is cooked. Keep the lid on until ready to serve.

Basmati Rice

1 Tbs. oil   1 cup rice   1 1/4 cup water

Heat the oil in a pan. Add rice and stir constantly until light brown. Then add water and cook at medium heat for 15 minutes or until cooked.

Fried Rice (brown or basmati)

2 cups cooked rice   1 tsp. salt
2 Tbs. oil   1/2 tsp. cayenne pepper
1 tsp. mustard seeds   if desired
1 small chopped onion   1/2 tsp. turmeric
1/4 to 1/2 chopped green pepper

Heat oil in a pan. Add mustard seeds. When they pop add onion and green pepper. Cook for a few minutes and then add rice and spices. Cook again for a few minutes. Serves 2 or 3.

Pulao

3 Tbs. oil   1 cup green peas (fresh or
2 cups basmati rice   frozen)
4 cups water   1/4 cup raisins
1/4 chopped green pepper   1/4 cup chopped cashews
1 chopped carrot   1 1/2 tsp. salt

Heat oil in a pan. Add cumin seeds. When they turn brown add rice and stir constantly until light brown. Then add water and remaining ingredients. Cook at medium heat 15 to 20 minutes. Serves 5 to 6.

Pulao Variation

After pulao is cooked spread yogurt on the top and cover until ready to serve.

Khichadi
(Basmati rice & split mung beans)

1/2 cup split mung beans   1/4 tsp. fenugreek seeds
1/2 cup basmati rice   5-6 whole black peppers

1 1/2 cup water   1/2 tsp. turmeric
1 Tbs. oil   1/2 tsp. salt
1/2 tsp. mustard seeds

This can be cooked in the pressure cooker the same as brown
rice, or use the following instructions:
Mix beans and rice in a container, wash twice and drain. In a
separate pan heat oil and add mustard seeds, fenugreek, and
black pepper. When the seeds pop add turmeric and washed rice
and bean mixture. Then add water and salt. Cook at medium
heat for 15-20 minutes.
Variation: You can add chopped onions after the mixture begins
to boil.

Khichadi
(Brown rice & whole mung beans)

1/2 cup brown rice   1/2 tsp. cumin seeds
1/2 cup mung beans   1/2 tsp. turmeric
2 cups water   1/2 tsp. salt
1 Tbs. oil

Mix rice and beans in a container, rinse twice. Add water and
salt. In a tiny container add oil and cumin seeds. When it turns
brown add turmeric. Add this to the rice and bean mixture.
Cook in a pressure cooker the same as brown rice.

BREADS

Spicy Bhakhari

2 cups whole wheat flour   1/2 tsp. ground black
6 Tbs. oil   pepper
1 tsp. salt   1 tsp. cumin seed powder
1/2 tsp. turmeric   1/2 cup water
1/2 tsp. cayenne pepper   soya oil for shallow
                                                   frying

Add oil and all spices to the flour and mix well. Add water
making the dough. Prepare about 12 balls. Flatten between

palms and then roll with rolling pin on a wooden board into 6" rounds.

Heat a thick flat pan. Cook the rolled bhakhari for 30 seconds on both sides at low heat. Add 1/4 tsp. oil, press with a spoon and cook on both sides until slightly brown.

Plain bhakhari: Same as above using only flour, oil, and water.

Puri (spicy)

2 cups whole wheat flour	1/2 tsp. black pepper
7 Tbs. oil	1 tsp. cumin seed powder
1 tsp. salt	1/2 cup water
1/2 tsp. turmeric	soya oil for deep frying
1/2 tsp. cayenne pepper	(about 2 cups)

Prepare the dough the same as spicy bhakhari. Make about 30 small balls and flatten them between palms. Then roll on a wooden board into 3" rounds.

Heat oil in a deep frying pan. Put two puris in at a time. When they puff, turn them over until cooked. Remove with a slotted spoon.

Plain puri Same as above using flour, oil, salt and water only.

Chopda

1 cup whole wheat flour	5 oz. water
3 Tbs. oil	Extra oil in a small bowl
1/2 tsp. salt	Extra flour in a small bowl

Mix flour, oil and salt. Then add water to make dough. Shape into 6 round balls and flatten between palms. Roll on a wooden board making 6" rounds.

Spread 1/8 tsp. oil on chopda, fold in half, add 1/8 tsp. oil and fold into fourths. Sprinkle flour on both sides and roll again. Cook both sides on a thick flat pan the same as bhakhari.

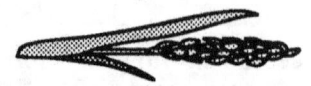

VEGETABLES

Vegetables can be prepared two ways: They can be stir-fried in oil to make them crisp, or cooked in water to make them soft and soupy.

STIR-FRIED VEGETABLES

The following vegetables or combinations can be cooked in oil:

Potatoes	Mixed vegetables
String beans	Cabbage and green peas
String beans and potatoes	Cauliflower and potatoes

Potatoes I

3 medium potatoes	1 tsp. salt
3 Tbs. soya oil	1 Tbs. coriander powder
1/2 tsp. cumin seeds	1 tsp. sugar
1/2 tsp. mustard seeds	1 Tbs. lemon juice
1/2 tsp. turmeric	

Wash potatoes and cut into 1/4" cubes. In a shallow pan heat oil, mustard and cumin seeds. When they pop, add potatoes, salt, and turmeric. Cook at low heat 20 minutes with occasional stirring. Add remaining spices.

Potatoes II

2 large potatoes boiled, peeled	1 tsp. salt
and cut into 1/4" cubes	1 Tbs. sesame seeds
3 Tbs. oil	3 Tbs. chopped peanuts
1/2 tsp. cumin seeds	1 tsp. sugar
1/4 tsp. turmeric	2 Tbs. lemon juice

In a large frying pan, heat oil and cumin seeds. When they turn brown add all ingredients and mix well. Cook 2 to 3 minutes.

Mixed Vegetables

2 cups cut string beans
(frozen or fresh)
1/4 cup frozen lima beans
1 cup mixed vegetables
(corn, peas, carrots, broccoli)
2 Tbs. oil

1/2 tsp. mustard seeds
1/2 tsp. turmeric
1 tsp. salt
1 tsp. curry powder
1 Tbs. coriander
powder
2 Tbs. grated coconut

Heat the oil in a heavy pan. Add mustard seeds. When they pop add all vegetables, salt, and turmeric. Cook at low heat for 15 to 20 minutes. Then add all spices and cook a few more minutes.

SOUPY VEGETABLES

The following vegetables or combinations can be made into soupy vegetables:

eggplant and potatoes
pumpkin and string beans
zucchini and corn

fresh dill and eggplant
spinach and eggplant
tofu and vegetables

Eggplant and Potatoes

2 medium potatoes cut
into long slices
1 medium eggplant cut
into long slices
2 fresh chopped tomatoes
1 chopped onion
1/4 chopped green pepper
3 Tbs. soya oil

1 tsp. cumin seeds
1 tsp. salt
1/2 tsp. turmeric
1/2 tsp. curry powder
1 Tbs. coriander
3 Tbs. sugar
1 Tbs. grated coconut
1 cup water

Heat oil in medium sauce-pan. Add cumin seeds. When they turn brown, add potatoes and water. Cook for a few minutes then add remaining ingredients. Cook at medium heat for 10 minutes.

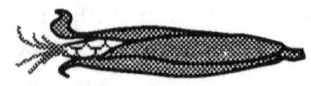

Zucchini and Corn

3 medium zucchini	1/2 tsp. salt
1 cup fresh or frozen corn	1/2 tsp. black pepper
2 Tbs. oil	1/2 tsp. cumin seed powder
1 tsp. cumin seeds	1 Tbs. lemon juice
	1 tsp. sugar

First peel zucchini and cut into 1/4" cubes. In a sauce-pan heat oil and cumin seeds. When they turn brown add zucchini and salt. Cook at low heat for 5 minutes. Then add corn and spices and cook 5 more minutes.

Tofu Vegetables

1/2 lb. tofu cut into 1/2" cubes	1/2 tsp. cumin seeds
5 choppped tomatoes	1 tsp. salt
1 chopped onion	1 tsp. curry powder
1/2 chopped green pepper	1/2 tsp. black pepper
1 cut potato	1 Tbs. sugar
2 Tbs. oil	2 cups water
	oil for frying

First fry the tofu in oil using deep frying pan until it turns brown. (You can saute it instead.)
In a sauce-pan heat oil and add cumin seeds. When they turn brown, add all vegetables and water and cook at medium heat. When vegetables are cooked add tofu and remaining spices. Cook 7 to 10 minutes.
If you want to make it more soupy add more water. Add arrowroot powder or any other thickener if you want it thicker.

CASSEROLES

Spinach Lasagna

10 oz. lasagna (artichoke or whole wheat)	1 lb. mashed tofu
	1/2 Tbs. salt
24 oz. frozen spinach or	1/2 tsp. black pepper
5 cups fresh chopped spinach	32 oz. tomato sauce

2 chopped onions	1 cup grated cheese
1/2 chopped green pepper	1 1/2 cup tomato sauce
	1 cup grated cheese

Add lasagna to boiling water. Cook 5 to 7 minutes. Drain. In a large container cook spinach, onions, green peppers for 5 minutes. After spinach is cooked add mashed tofu, cheese, salt and pepper. Turn off heat. Oil a 9" x 12" flat pan. Place (total of five layers) first layer of lasagna, then spinach mixture, repeat with a final layer of lasagna. Spread sauce and cheese over the top. Bake for 45 minutes at 350° F. Serves 8 to 10.

Spinach Casserole

1/2 package Fillo	1 Tbs. salt
24 oz. frozen spinach (or 5	1 tsp. black pepper
cups fresh chopped spinach)	16 oz. sour cream
2 chopped onions	2 cups grated cheese
1/2 green pepper	1/2 lb. melted butter
1/4 cup olive pieces	

Cook spinach, onion, and green pepper together, then add everything except butter. In a 9" x 12" flat pan, make five layers. First layer is 5 pieces of fillo, second is spinach mixture, repeat with a final layer of fillo. Pour melted butter on top. Bake at 350° F. for 30 minutes or until fillo turns slightly brown.

Zucchini Casserole

2 cups sliced zucchini	1 tsp. salt
2 cups sliced tomatoes	1/2 tsp. black pepper
1/2 chopped green pepper	1 tsp. oregano
2 medium chopped onions	1 cup grated cheese

First steam zucchini, onion, and pepper. In a casserole pan place a layer of half the zucchini followed by a tomato layer. Spread half of the spices on top followed by remaining zucchini. Spread grated cheese and remaining spices on top. Bake at 300 ° F for 20 minutes or until cheese melts.

Soya Bean Casserole

1 cup soya beans	1/2 cup fresh or frozen corn
2 cups water	1 tsp. salt
1 1/2 cup tomato sauce	3 tsp. oregano leaves
2 chopped onions	1 cup grated cheese
1/2 chopped green pepper	butter

Soak soya beans overnight and wash thoroughly in the morning. Cook soya beans 30 minutes in a pressure cooker with 2 cups water and salt.
Grease casserole pan with butter. Add cooked beans and spices. Sprinkle cheese on top. Bake at 350° F. 30 minutes or until cheese melts.

Broccoli and Cauliflower Casserole

4 cups steamed vegetables (broccoli, cauliflower, onion, green pepper)	1 tsp. oregano leaves
	1/2 tsp. black pepper or cayenne pepper
1/2 cup sour cream or yogurt	1 cup grated cheese
2 cups thick mushroom soup (canned)	butter or margarine

Butter the casserole pan. Add steamed vegetables and all ingredients except cheese and mix well. Spread cheese on top. Bake at 350° F. for 20 minutes.

SIDE DISHES

Upma

3 Tbs. soya oil   1/2 tsp. cumin seed   1 cup cream of wheat

Heat the oil in a thick sauce-pan. Add cumin seeds. When they turn brown add cream of wheat and stir constantly at medium heat for 5 minutes. Turn off heat.

3 Tbs. oil	2 cups water
3 Tbs. split chick peas or	1 cup buttermilk/yogurt
yellow split peas	1 tsp. salt
1/4 cup chopped carrots	3 Tbs. sugar
1/2 cup green peas	3 Tbs. lemon juice
1/4 chopped green pepper	1/2 tsp. ground black
	pepper

In another pan heat oil. Add split peas and stir. When it turns brown add all ingredients and boil. After it boils add cream of wheat mixture. Cook at low heat for 5 minutes or until water evaporates

Tabouli

3 Tbs. soya oil	1 stalk chopped celery
1 cup cracked or bulgar	1/2 green chopped pepper
wheat	1 tsp. salt
1 cup cooked or canned	1 tsp. cumin seed powder
chick peas	1 tsp. basil leaves
2 cups water	1/2 cup chopped peanut,
1 chopped carrot	cashew, sunflower mix
2 chopped onions	

Heat oil in a sauce-pan. Saute cracked wheat until brown. Then add everything and cook 20 minutes over low heat.

Falafill

Whole wheat pita bread	1 tsp. salt
2 cups chick peas	1 Tbs. garlic
	1 cup water

Soak chick peas overnight. Wash thoroughly and then blend in blender with water. Add garlic and salt.
Heat oil in a deep frying pan. Make one inch round balls of chick pea mixture and place in pan. Fry until golden brown.

Falafill Sauce

1/2 bunch chopped parsley	3 Tbs. lemon juice
1 tsp. salt	4 Tbs. oil
1 tsp. black pepper	1 cup chopped lettuce
1/2 tsp. cayenne pepper	3/4 cup water

Blend all ingredients in a blender. Cut the pita in half to make pocket bread. Place sauce, chick pea balls, chopped lettuce, tomatoes, sprouts, etc. in pocket.

Sprouted Mung Beans

2 cups sprouted mung beans
2 Tbs. oil
1/2 tsp. cumin seeds
1 tsp. salt

1/2 tsp. turmeric
1 tsp. sugar
1 Tbs. grated coconut
2 Tbs. lemon juice
1/4 chopped green pepper

Steam mung beans 3 to 5 minutes. In a medium sauce-pan heat oil and add cumin seeds. When they turn brown add mung beans and all spices. Cook at low heat for 5 minutes.

Tofu Sauce

1 lb. tofu-mashed
1 bunch chopped parsley
1 Tbs. salt
3 Tbs. lemon juice

2 Tbs. chopped garlic
1/2 cup sunflower seeds
1 1/2 cups water

Blend everything in a blender until it turns into sauce. Use as a salad dressing or sandwich spread.

Yogurt

2 cups milk

1/4 cup plain yogurt or buttermilk

Heat milk to boiling. Leave at room temperature to cool. When slightly warm add yogurt and stir. Let it sit in a warm place without disturbance for 12 to 18 hours. Then keep in refrigerator for one day.

Indian Tea

1 cup water
1 cup milk
2 Tbs. sugar

1/4 tsp. tea spices
8 to 10 fresh mint leaves
3 to 4 tea bags

Mix everything and boil for a few minutes. Tea spices are available in an Indian or health food store (Yogi tea). You can eliminate tea bags and sugar or substitute for them.

Cucumber Raita

1 cup grated peeled cucumber
1 cup plain yogurt
1/2 cup sour cream
1 tsp. salt
2 tsp. sugar

1 tsp. cumin seed
powder
1 Tbs. mustard seed powder
1/2 tsp. ground black pepper
1/4 cup raisins
1/8 cup chopped cashews

Mix cucumber and salt and let it sit for 5 minutes. Then squeeze out all water. Add remaining ingredients and mix.

Carrot Raita

1 cup grated carrots

Follow the directions for cucumber raita using same ingredients and add carrots.

Eggplant Raita

2 cups eggplant cut into
1/4 inch pieces
1/2 cup water
1 Tbs. oil
1/2 tsp. cumin seeds

1 tsp. salt
1/2 tsp. cumin seed powder
1/2 tsp. black pepper
1 tsp. salt
1 cup yogurt

Heat the oil in a pan, then add cumin seeds. When they turn brown add eggplant and spices. Cover and cook on low heat for 7 to 10 minutes. Sit until cool and then add yogurt.

Pizza

3/4 cup whole wheat flour
3/4 cup unbleached
white flour
6 oz. warm water

1 cup tomato sauce
1 chopped onion
1/4 cup chopped green
pepper

1 Tbs. baking yeast	1 cup grated cheese
1/2 tsp. salt	oil and flour
2 Tbs. oil	

Soak yeast in warm water for 15 minutes. Then add both flours, salt and oil and prepare the dough. Cover and leave it in a warm place for 1/2 hour or until it rises.

Knead the dough using some oil. Then make a big round ball, cover it with some flour, and roll it on a flat form.

In a pizza dish spread 1 Tbs. oil and 1 tsp. flour. Transfer the rolled dough to the pizza dish and spread it to cover the dish. Then spread sauce, green pepper and onion (or add any other topping as desired) followed by grated cheese.

Bake at 450° F. for 30 to 40 minutes or until cooked.

Note: You may use soya mozzarella instead of regular cheese.

S W E E T S

Mixed Nut Candy

3 Tbs. sweet butter or ghee	1/2 cup sunflower
1 1/2 cup brown sugar	seeds
1/2 cup sesame seeds	1/2 cup chopped peanuts
	1/2 cup chopped cashews

In a thick cast iron pan melt the butter. Then add brown sugar and stir constantly at medium heat until it starts to bubble. Next add all nuts and mix well. Turn off the heat. Spread the mixture on a wooden board or a flat buttered dish. Cut it when warm.

Shikhand I

8 oz. cream cheese	pinch of saffron
2 cups plain yogurt	1 tsp. ground cardamon
2 cups sour cream	powder
1 1/2 cups sugar	1/4 cup chopped almonds

In a sauce-pan put cream cheese and sugar and let it sit at room temperature to soften. Then beat it with an electric mixer until all

lumps are broken and the mixture is uniform. Add remaining ingredients and mix. Cool in refrigerator before serving.
Note: Use less sugar if desired.

Shikhand II

64 oz. plain yogurt   1 tsp. cardamon powder
(two 32 oz. containers)   pinch of saffron
1 1/2 cup sugar   1/4 cup chopped almonds

Place yogurt in a cheesecloth or cotton cloth to drain all water from the yogurt (5 hours). Place the drained yogurt in a container. Add all ingredients and mix with an electric mixer.

Fruit Salad I

3 cups milk   1 cup canteloup
1 cup half and half   1 tsp. cardamon
2 bananas   1/4 tsp. saffron
3 peeled apples   1/2 cup sugar
1 cup chopped watermelon   1 tsp. nutmeg
     2 Tbs. grated coconut

Warm the milk in a large container and then cool. Cut all fruits into small pieces. Place fruit in the cooled milk. Add remaining ingredients and mix. Cool in the refrigerator before serving.

Fruit Salad II

1 banana   1/2 cup fresh pineapple
1 apple   1 peeled orange
2 peaches   1/2 cup raisins
1 cup chopped watermelon   1/2 cup chopped cashews
1/2 cup canteloup   2 Tbs. coconut
1/2 cup honeydew   1/4 cup sunflower seeds
1/2 cup grapes

Cut all fruits and mix in a large container. (You can use any fruits in season.) Add remaining ingredients and mix. Refrigerate before serving.

Rasmalai

16 oz. ricotta cheese	1/2 tsp. cardamon powder
1 cup dry milk powder	5 chopped almonds
1/2 cup sugar	warm sweet butter

Mix all the ingredients. Butter a flat dish and spread the mixture making 1/4" layer (may take two pizza dishes). Bake at 300° F. for 30 minutes or until top becomes slightly brown. Cool.
While it is cooking warm the following mixture in a separate container and cool.

4 cups milk	pinch of saffron
1 cup half and half	1 tsp. nutmeg
3/4 cup sugar	5 chopped almonds

Cut the baked mixture into small square pieces and add to the cold milk mixture. Cool in refrigerator. Serves 8 to 10.

Baklava

1/2 package of fillo	1 tsp. cardamon
1 cup chopped walnuts	1/2 cup sugar
1 cup chopped cashews	1/4 cup coconut
1/2 cup raisins	1/2 cup warm sweet butter
Syrup:	
1 cup sugar	
2 cups water	

Mix all nuts, sugar and spices. In a 9" x 12" flat container place 5 pieces of fillo then spread nut mix, repeat and top with a final layer of fillo (5 layers in all). Spread warm butter on top and bake at 300° F. for 25 minutes or until top turns golden brown. Cool.
In a sauce-pan heat sugar and water. Boil 5 to 7 minutes. Cool. Pour cooled syrup on top of cooled baklava mixture. Cut into squares.

Shiro

1/2 cup warm sweet butter	3/4 cup sugar
3/4 cup cream of wheat	1 tsp. cardamon powder
15 raisins	8 chopped almonds
1 1/2 cup water or milk	

Melt butter in sauce-pan and add cream of wheat. Cook at medium heat with constant stirring until light brown. Then add raisins and mix. Add water or milk and cook with occasional stirring until water or milk has evaporated. Add sugar and stir constantly for 5 minutes. Turn off heat and add cardamon and almonds. Mix and serve. Or, spread the mixture on a flat dish and cut into squares.

Sweet Cracked Wheat

2 cups water	1 tsp. nutmeg
1 cup sugar	15 raisins
1 Tbs. grated coconut	1 cup cracked wheat
1/2 tsp. cardamon	3 Tbs. sweet warm butter

Mix all ingredients except cracked wheat and butter in a pan and boil. Then add cracked wheat and butter. Turn off heat. Transfer this mixture to a small container and then to a pressure cooker containing 1 1/2 cups water. Cook 10 to 15 minutes.

Notes: People on a macrobiotic diet may modify by eliminating sugar and tomatoes. Sugar can be substituted with unrefined natural sugar, raw or brown sugar, brown rice syrup, barley malt, or solid Indian molasses.

GUIDANCE

25. Seven Week Yoga Course

26. Daily Practice Routine

27. Daily Influence of Yoga

28. Affirmations

29. Daily Affirmations

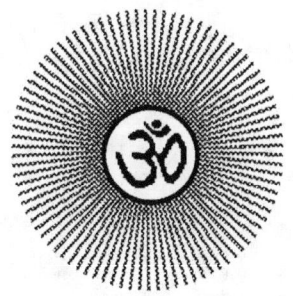

25

SHANTI YOGA INSTITUTE

SEVEN WEEK HATHA YOGA COURSE

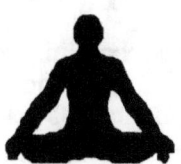

This course is designed for individuals or groups. Classes meet once a week for one hour or more. Each session includes a review of postures introduced the previous week. Appropriate reading assignments are given for each lesson and classes include time for discussions and questions.

1. General introduction to Yoga. Waking up properly, basic stretching and limbering. Neck and eye rotations, arms and legs stretching, palming, cow's head, leg lift, rocking. Head-to-knee, cobra, simple twist, preparation for sitting positions. Abdominal breathing and relaxation.

2. Rotation around the waist, greeting behind the back, swan. Half lotus, squatting, boat on back, bow, forward bending standing. Yogic breathing and relaxation. Introduction to diet.

3. Eagle, shoulderstand, plough, fish, Yoga mudra, camel, stork. Introduction to fasting. Cleansing breathing and third eye concentration.

4. Combination shoulderstand/plough/bridge/fish routine, twist variation, dundasana. Prana and healing discussion. Cleansing techniques. Healing breathing and relaxation.

5. Introduction to sun prayer. Head-to-knee variations, triangle, lotus, stomach press, half headstand. Rhythmic breathing, relaxation.

6. Sun prayer, complete shoulderstand routine with variations, locust, chest expander, lion, and stomach lift. Recharging breathing and relaxation.

7. Complete stretching and limbering routine. Shoulderstand routine, boat on stomach, twist on back, forward/backward bending routine. Introduction of arrow shooting, nauli, and advanced breathing and meditation techniques. Guidance for setting up daily routine.

A car is traveling at a slower speed in a drizzle. When it picks up speed it seems as if the rain is coming down harder. When we evolve faster, we face more adversities in life.

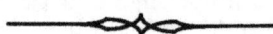

We should not feel guilty when we enjoy life. It is good to enjoy our creation of art, beauty, and accomplishments. This joy expands and frees us and gives us self-confidence. Holding onto joy is attachment. Dwelling mentally, thinking, worrying, or daydreaming is attachment.

Spiritual life and spiritual disciplines should not make you serious and gloomy. They should make you innocent and childlike, having fun in life. They should allow you to have innocent laughs and jokes and to treat life as a play.

26

DAILY PRACTICE ROUTINE

Follow the <u>General Rules and Preparation for Hatha Yoga</u> in Chapter 4. Practice the routine of Yoga positions and meditation regularly twice a day as explained below. If time does not permit, follow the mini routine, or modify the regular one to suit your schedule and personal needs.

PART 1

ROUTINE OF YOGA POSITIONS
(Complete Routine)

1. Stretching and warm-up:
   Neck roll, rocking, stretching arms and legs, swan, sun prayer.

2. Headstand (optional) for 1 to 3 minutes.
   Rest on the back for 1 minute. (Do this only if you have been taught properly.)

3. Shoulderstand Routine:
   Shoulderstand - 1 to 3 minutes
   Plough-bridge-fish (30 seconds each)
   Rocking to relax the back, rest for 2 minutes with abdominal breathing.

4. Forward bending posture:
   Head-to-knee with or without variations. Two times, hold 30 seconds.

5. Backward bending posture:
   Bow - two times, retain for 30 seconds.

6. Twist position - one time in each direction, 30 second retention.

7. Lion - two or three times.

8.   Abdominal Lift - two or three rounds.

9.   Balancing Position: Balance on each leg one time each, retain comfortably.

10.   Miscellaneous Positions: Do these as a challenge and for learning new positions or new variations.

11.   Corpse Position, Breathing and Relaxation
        (See Chapter 7, Relaxation.)

PART 2

BREATHING AND MEDITATION ROUTINE

        Practice this routine in the beginning, middle, or at the end of your Yoga Position program to suit your needs.

1.   Practice one or more of the following breathing techniques and meditation:

        A. Yogic breathing followed by Rhythmic or Recharging Breathing.

        B. Cleansing Breathing followed by Third Eye concentration or Heart Center meditation.

        C. Anuloma Viloma Pranayama (Alternate Nostril Breathing) followed by SO HUM meditation.

2.   Chant OM aloud three to ten times, and then mentally
                            or
        Chant the Guru Mantra followed by OM chant-first aloud, whispered, and then mentally.

3.   Read any inspiring paragraph from this book (or any scriptural reading), a General Affirmation (See page 240.) followed by one of the Daily Affirmations. (See Chapter 29.)

MINI ROUTINE

1. Practice some stretching exercises to allow the body to be relaxed and comfortable.

2. Practice Cleansing Breathing following by any meditation technique to suit your needs.

3. Go through total shoulderstand routine.

4. Relax on your back with Recharging Breathing.

5. Read one of the Daily Affirmations from Chapter 29.

DAILY DISCIPLINES

1. Be regular in sleeping and waking. (Wake up early.)

2. Eat moderately at regular times and with awareness.

3. Be moderate in your actions by balancing physical and mental activities.

4. Go through the daily morning cleansing techniques as explained in Chapter 23, Cleansing.

5. Read from scriptures or an inspirational portion of this book.

6. Associate with positive friends, avoid negative environment. During the day become aware of your thoughts, words, activities, and breathing patterns. Chant a mantra aloud or mentally whenever possible.

7. Be flexible with your disciplines and enjoy life. Smile, laugh, and be free.

GENERAL DISCIPLINES

1. Once a week fast for twenty-four hours on juice, fruits, or water. Use this day for meditation and introspection.

2. Practice a longer fast two to four times a year along with an internal cleansing program.

3. Try to become a vegetarian. Reduce your consumption of meat, alcohol, stimulants, junk food, etc.

4. Maintain weekly contact with a Yoga class, group association, or friends to recharge your spiritual life.

We should digest ideas and inspirations that come from other souls. Each of us has a different temperament, different tendencies and constitutions depending on our birth, upbringing, and experiences of life, due to our Karma. Imitation is only a show. Each great soul had a unique personal experience which is reflected in his life through different behavior. Imitating this behavior does not give us any glimpse of truth.

Conserve time, money, and energy. These are the requirements for material or spiritual success. Channel this energy in the desired direction. One drop of water at a time cuts rocks and will fill an ocean.

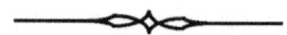

Some people become more attached to life and fear death as they grow older. Thus they suffer in proportion to their attachments. We can grow in wisdom as we age. The choice is ours.

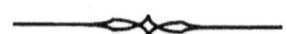

27

DAILY INFLUENCE OF YOGA

Our total being operates in unity where the body, breath, senses, and mind are interconnected. The body itself is an integrated unit of muscles, organs, glands, and nerves. Since everything is interconnected, we cannot treat one area of the body to eliminate a specific problem; rather we must work with our entire body, senses, and mind to bring about the required balance. If a specific "problem" is treated by drugs, not realizing that the drugs only act on the symptoms of the problem, only suppression or temporary relief will be found. However, to heal our total being we must take responsibility for our life and, with patience and perseverance, cultivate a holistic approach.

The Yoga program is designed for preventive maintenance and the elimination of basic health problems. We recommend the daily routine as described in Chapter 26, and you will experience the benefits described in this chapter in a natural way. Each person is different and will not respond at the same rate or to the same degree. A person with many abnormalities will notice quicker results due to clear contrasts. A young and healthy person will need to be more aware of subtle changes. He will be building up preventive measures of health for future years. Progress in Yoga is measured from where you begin. Even if you have inherited a weak body or begin at a later stage in life, you will notice that you enjoy greater health benefits with the practice of Yoga. You should not compare yourself with anyone, nor should you push yourself. Pushing will only produce strain and frustration. Learn to love and accept yourself and become your own friend.

People with physical handicaps or limitations can always practice some aspect of Yoga. They can practice breathing or meditation, or read while bedridden or sick. One should focus on what he can do and let that begin the chain reaction of a positive life style and avoid worrying about things he cannot do.

Yoga practice should be enjoyable and not a chore. You practice not because you have to and it is good for you, but because you love to do it. In time you will look forward to this personal time just for yourself.

Practice with eyes closed and be aware of the deep muscles as you stretch them. As you do this, tensions will drain out of your body. Deep emotional scars of your life and traumatic experiences which are locked in the deep muscles will be released; you will experience lightness of body and mind. You will gain closer contact with your inner being and deeper feelings instead of hiding away from them in the form of restless activities in the world. As burdens are removed you will feel happy; your total being will express this happiness, and people around you will notice and remark about it. This should encourage you to keep up with your practice. If you go for a medical check up, your doctor will be surprised at the positive changes in your health. Your inner feeling of security will attract people towards you, seeking your company and advice.

If you have been engaged in sports, distance running, dancing, aerobics, weight lifting, etc. you will discover that yogic breathing, rhythm and awareness become integrated into your other disciplines. You will enjoy them more by removing the competitive aspects and making them more meditative. Yoga will be so satisfying that the need for other exercises will be reduced. Yoga provides all cardiovascular benefits without shocking your heart, injuring your joints or muscles, heavy breathing, oxygen starvation, sweating, or muscle soreness.

As the body stretches and becomes flexible you experience youthfulness and enthusiasm for life. Flexibility in the body brings flexibility to the mind. The mind becomes open, receptive, tolerant, and creative. These qualities bring success in life. As postures and breathing improve you feel more positive, assertive, alert and are in a position to communicate and influence others. Yoga practices balance the body and mind. For example, if one leg is longer than the other the rest of the body tries to compensate creating further imbalance. Yoga balances the body by removing the imbalance. By practicing balancing with concentration you activate the left (logical) and right (intuition) sides of the brain bringing them together so you coordinate logic and intuition in normal daily situations.

As the stomach and other internal organs are exercised you improve digestion, metabolism, and elimination. Improved breathing helps in the oxidation of food. These factors together help burn calories and sustain a stable, healthy weight.

With regular Yoga practice the body becomes firm, flabbiness disappears, and weight is adjusted and balanced properly. Thyroid and parathyroid glands are balanced and normalized, resulting in normal body weight. Excess weight comes off and people having a problem gaining will increase their weight. In other words, optimum weight for individual body structure, constitution, height and age, is secured with regular Yoga practice. As this occurs, you feel comfortable and happy. The body's built-in buffer system holds weight within five pounds regardless of intake. One should be happy with this and not push himself to attain a standard weight from height-weight charts, or models set by society or TV commercials.

As one exercises the total body, receiving a proper oxygen supply and quieting the mind with meditation, one feels content and peaceful. His body will choose a proper diet, rejecting meat, junk food, overeating, stimulants, alcohol and drugs, and he will enjoy a healthy, balanced diet. One becomes aware of his body as a temple of God and respects it. He will not hurt or punish himself by smoking, drinking, wrong eating or sleeping habits. Breathing will satisfy the lungs and increase one's awareness of each activity. This proper breathing weakens the urge for smoking as well as eliminates impulsive habits and behavior which are done without awareness.

Yoga stimulates all the vital organs so they eliminate toxins from the body by means of sweating, exhaling carbon dioxide, proper elimination; the body functions efficiently like a well tuned car. One finds more energy during the day, rejuvenates real hunger, and sleeps better. Headaches caused by tension or a clogged body are eliminated and insomnia is removed; one wakes up refreshed.

Yoga provides mastery of Self. Practicing Yoga positions helps the joints, reduces arthritic conditions, strengthens the back, reduces backaches, improves circulation, strengthens the heart, and normalizes blood pressure. After mastering the art of breathing one can control the mind, and eliminate disturbing emotions and stress. By maintaining calmness of mind one increases immunity against disease. With meditation and attunement one connects his mind with vital functions of the body and establishes a biofeedback response which helps control heart, lungs, breathing, and stressful situations.

Emotional balance is attained naturally. One maintains evenness of mind and rises above mood swings.

Creative energy is preserved and one naturally loses attachment for trivial things. Petty situations don't disturb his peace and he can focus on the important spiritual issues of life.

One naturally feels attracted toward a spiritual environment and friends, and loses interest in restless activities such as parties and wrong associations. His life becomes simple, goals become clear, and he becomes an inspiration to those around him.

All of the above benefits are real and will come to you in time. However, effort and diligent practice are required.

We don't need to go out in the world to provide service. If we look around we find many situations where we can provide service . Ignoring our basic duties and going out to serve others is escapism.

Ask, am I serving out of love, compassion, and with non-attachment or out of self-pity, reward, and ego? The former will provide freedom and joy; the latter will produce stress and exhaustion.

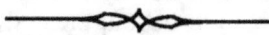

First think, then speak and act. This process gives integration of personality, peace, and harmony. Disharmony is in proportion to the distance between thoughts, words, and deeds. Compulsive behavior begins from action - e.g., gambling, smoking, buying, then the mind and speech try to justify action. This defensive attitude wastes energy.

The less you talk the more prana power will flow through your words, conveying conviction, strength, and appeal. Useless waste of words dilutes this energy. Lying, gossiping, exaggerations, and dry intellectual talk drain energy.

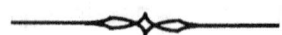

28

AFFIRMATIONS

What are Affirmations?

Affirmations are certain phrases with deep positive meanings which are recited or thought about and make a deep impression on the mind to bring about positive changes in life.

Process of Affirmation

We exist in three bodies: Physical, Astral, and Causal. These three bodies exist concurrently. We use one or more of the above bodies in combination, depending upon activity and spiritual evolution.

Gross Body: The gross body comprises our physical structure. It is made of flesh and bones, organs of action, and five senses. This body, held together by prana, is used during normal conscious activities.

Astral Body: The astral body comprises the mind and intellect. This body is used when we think, dream, or daydream. The subconscious and unconscious states are part of this body.

Causal Body: This body is used in the transcendental state during meditation and dreamless sleep.

We constantly absorb ideas, suggestions, and feelings from our environment by using all three bodies. All impressions are communicated among these bodies depending upon the intensity of the experience.

Physical

During the waking state, the body and senses absorb impressions. For example: watching TV, reading, talking, tasting, touching, smelling, etc. These impressions are registered in the mind. Intense and prolonged exposure to any environment produces longer lasting impressions. These impressions are recalled and brought to the surface by proper stimulation or by free will.

The gross body follows the laws of matter: i.e., physics, weight, volume, density, etc.

Astral

Our astral body is activated when we think. During the day and during sleep we unknowingly fall into a semi-hypnotic state where thoughts and impressions are strongly registered without our conscious knowledge. From early childhood we are constantly being brainwashed into different beliefs. These deep impressions control our life to a greater extent than our conscious mental control.

Impressions are picked up by infants as well as by unborn babies. The unborn baby is influenced by the food the mother eats, by her thoughts, and by her emotions. An unconscious person under anesthesia or in a coma picks up all the impressions with his astral body.

The astral body adheres to the subtle and powerful laws of mind and psychic laws. The power of astral projection, clairvoyance, clairaudience, telepathy, etc., are examples of man's ability to rise above the laws of physics. The intuitive faculty absorbs knowledge without the presence of the senses.

Causal

If we meditate regularly and maintain spiritual awareness, we reach the causal state. This is a transcendental state where one is aware of "I Am", without body, mind, desires, size, shape, likes, dislikes, etc. One bypasses the laws of physics and psychics, and tunes into cosmic energy. At this level, spiritual laws exist and miracles are produced. When we reach this level all of our needs are fulfilled. We don't need to ask for anything. Spirit knows it all.

Causal level is the source of all energy. This energy extends to the astral level, and from there it reaches the gross level of our existence. It is similar to the powerful heat and light of the sun reaching the moon, and the moon's faint light being reflected onto the earth.

The causal body is the roots; astral body is the trunk and branches, while the gross body is the leaves, flowers, and fruits. We should nurture the roots of positive affirmations and destroy the roots of negative impressions in order to reap the reward of sweet fruits in our lives. For best results, we should treat our total personality instead of treating the body alone.

Affirmations and the Life Force

In terms of Yoga, affirmation means using thoughts to direct prana, the life force. All healings are produced by this life force. We can learn to direct prana to heal ourselves and others, as explained in Chapter 6, Breathing. This force can penetrate any space, and bring absentee healing. Everyone possesses and can cultivate this healing energy. Each thought and emotion changes the flow of prana which, in turn, changes our body chemistry. In a physical sense we can notice that thoughts and feelings bring about instantaneous changes in our body chemistry. For example, when you hear unpleasant shocking news, you interfere with the flow of prana; the supply is reduced which makes one weak and vulnerable and susceptible to negative influences. Your heart and lungs become irregular, tears come from your eyes, your stomach cramps, and you lose your appetite. Many other and less noticeable symptoms occur.

Such shocks and emotions lower our level of immunity and we become subject to disease and infection. Calmness of mind and positive experiences can bring about positive changes in our body chemistry by increasing the flow and rhythm of prana throughout our body.

Our body chemistry changes constantly as our emotions change. Research has proven that positive thoughts, beliefs, and affirmations produce secretion of hormones which increase immunity in the body. Certain hormones, called endorphins, can be secreted which produce euphoria and thus act as a pain killer. For example, if someone is in pain due to an injury, he inhibits the pain when a loved one visits him, when he thinks about some pleasant experience, or when he listens to pleasant music.

Thoughts Produce Chain Reactions

One positive thought will start a chain of positive thoughts. One negative thought will generate negative patterns of thoughts. If a person who has an illness can feel positive and experience love, endorphins will be produced which will suppress pain in a natural way. In the absence of pain, he will feel interested in life and can visualize or imagine pleasure and excitement, and his body will heal quickly.

On the other hand, a person who dwells on pain will magnify the pain and will imagine all the other diseases he is going to get. He may visualize the suffering of others that he has seen in the past and thereby attract suffering to himself to his own self-destruction. He also unconsciously picks up negative remarks from others including doctors.

We have the choice of producing a thought body through positive or negative thoughts. This thought body, accompanied by visualization and imagination, becomes reality. The thoughts precipitate and make it a material reality. At this time it can be treated physically. When it becomes chronic, it becomes hard to believe it could have been created by the mind.

We create or manufacture diseases and illnesses in our body. If we hang onto any emotional shock, guilt, resentment, anger, or fear, we only nurture the disease. It can manifest as cancer, a cold, arthritis, or heart problems, depending upon where and how we hold the tension. The moment we let go and start the positive direction of love, we release the disease.

When affirmations are made in a quiet state of mind they reach the astral and causal levels. These deep centers of our convictions become reality. Affirmations without belief in them, or affirmations that remain on the surface, merely become wishful thinking.

Preparation

1. Choose a comfortable room, a proper time and environment so you are completely open and at ease. Practice in the morning before starting your day, and at night before going to sleep.

2. Practice some Yoga positions or Yoga stretching exercises to free the body from tension.

3. Choose any suitable yogic breathing to quiet the mind and senses. Close your eyes.

4. Empty your mind of all thoughts. Let go of all the limitations created by your mind. Let go of all attachments: material, emotional, etc. Send forgiveness to all who have offended you. Send prayers of love to everyone in the world until you feel open and released.

5. Feel yourself a channel for God's energy.

6. Read the affirmations aloud, very slowly, and one line at a time in order to influence your gross body. Keep repeating them more and more softly until your voice becomes a whisper and then mental, to influence the astral body. At this point visualize with closed eyes and repeat mentally adding faith and conviction to the affirmation. Charge it with you prana, your soul energy, and add your emotions until you can believe in it as reality. This influences the causal body.

7. During the day dwell on the essence of your affirmation. Nurture it with the proper environment. Avoid people, situations, and talk which generate doubts or which neutralize the power of affirmations.

We need to learn to swim and learn life saving techniques before jumping into the water to save a drowning person. We need to grow spiritually before helping others. We must save ourselves before saving the world.

———◇———

Time cures grief. To overcome grief travel into the future mentally. The intensity of the grief will be reduced as time is speeded up mentally.

———◇———

Make it a habit to laugh every day by seeing, reading, or remembering some humorous event. Laughter will stimulate vital energy, speed the healing process, stimulate vital organs, and will allow you to free yourself from depression or negative emotions.

———◇———

Moderation is the key to meditation. Harsh disciplines or indulgences place a strain on life and destroy the joy of life.

———◇———

GENERAL AFFIRMATIONS

I accept myself.
I love myself.
I love life.

I thank God for the gifts of life - for human birth - a sound body and mind - for five organs of action: hands, feet, speech, excretion, reproduction. For five organs of perception: seeing, hearing, tasting, touching, smelling. For food and shelter, and friends and loved ones.

I accept these gifts as privileges and enjoy them fully from moment to moment without holding onto them, without attachment or expectation.

I take responsibility for all situations in my life.

I believe in the Law of Justice (Karma). What I deserve will be attracted to me.

I face the problems in life as challenges to teach me spiritual lessons.

I am willing to change and to make sacrifices to bring about these changes.

I am willing to dig deeper into my mind and face unpleasant suppressed emotions with a passive mind. These emotional patterns were established by parents, teachers, church, society, and myself.

I forgive everyone including myself and feel relief and freedom to experience the true reality of Self.

I am never alone. The Lord always looks after me.

The Lord is my guide and companion. I choose to come out of isolation so I can receive and give love unconditionally.

I am created in the image of God. I am a reflection of God. Perfection is my essential nature. Health, harmony, and prosperity are my birthright.

I deserve happiness, peace, prosperity, and harmony.

29

DAILY AFFIRMATIONS

DAY 1 - PURE EXISTENCE - SAT

I choose to quiet my body, senses, and mind and allow my spiritual heart to open up. Within the heart I feel the presence of Atman (Self), the real Me, the spark of Divine.

I am pure existence. I am omnipresent. I am within and without.

I was, I am, and I will be. I was never born and I will never die.

Time, space, cause, or effect do not bind me. Fire cannot burn me, water cannot drown me. Weapons cannot destroy me, robbers cannot rob me.

My body is only a vehicle. Changes in the body don't affect me. My mind is only my vehicle. Thoughts and emotions don't affect me.

I am perfect. I am wholesome. I am the Reality.

I have no goals because I am the Goal.

I have nothing to do, and nowhere to go.

I am the subject without any objects.

I will recharge myself during the day from time to time by tuning into my immortal Self to rise above limitations and fears.

I AM THAT I AM

DAY 2 - PURE CONSCIOUSNESS - CHIT

As I sit quietly, I become aware of the pure light of consciousness shining like a luminous sun within my heart. I am the spark of cosmic consciousness. I am omniscient.

All knowledge comes from my inner center.

I witness and transcend waking consciousness, dream consciousness, and the dreamless state of consciousness.

I am the witness of body, senses, thoughts, and emotions.

I let this inner consciousness reflect throughout my being.

I let this consciousness lead me to truth, and protect me from untruth.

I let this consciousness lead me to the light of wisdom and protect me from the darkness of ignorance.

I let this consciousness lead me to immortality and protect me from attachment to mortality.

I let this consciousness open my third eye of intuition which guides my way on the journey of life.

I choose to be aware during the day to witness my thoughts, emotions, speech, and actions without being involved in them.

I choose to rise above the limitations of dogma, religion, nationality, so the whole universe becomes my home.

I choose to maintain awareness that I am pure consciousness without age, sex, or status, and I experience the same divine spark of consciousness which is in all living creatures.

During the day I shall tune into my innermost reservoir for recharging myself.

DAY 3 - PURE BLISS - ANAND

As I become quiet I withdraw into my inner self. I let the gates of my heart open up and enter and experience the real abode of my being. I bathe in this inner reservoir of bliss, peace, and contentment.

I let this bliss, peace, and contentment radiate, expand, and saturate my body, senses, and mind. I allow it to flow into space to reach all living creatures until I experience homogeneous existence with the universe.

I let my life and its activities radiate the feeling of bliss which protects me from the transient and illusive happiness of the world.

My inner bliss will shine like a luminous light which burns all the dark sorrows of the world and fulfills all my desires

I will maintain awareness during the day and will recharge myself by tuning into my inner reservoir of peace when worldly ambitions, restlessness, and problems attack me.

I will reflect my spiritual joy with smiles, sweet speech, gestures, and actions to spread this joy everywhere I go.

DAY 4 - LOVE

As I become quiet, I experience the feeling of love deep within my heart. God reflects His presence within my heart in the form of Divine Love.

Divine Love is fulfilling, satisfying, and expanding. I let this love fill my heart, my mind, my senses, and my body. I allow this love to dissolve the restlessness of my mind and insecurities.

I let this love extend to all living creatures unconditionally until it saturates my consciousness. This ocean of love will dissolve all conflicts. I will experience deep healing and rejuvenation as love dissolves deep-rooted feelings of anger, hate, and resentments.

During the day I will chant the Lord's name with each breath. Chanting His name will keep the flame of love and surrender alive.

I will love my family and friends more unconditionally, accept them as they are, and forgive them.

I shall remember the Lord during the day when problems, attachments, desires, and confusion overwhelm me. I shall assert <u>Thy will be done and not mine.</u>

I will let my love radiate around me like the fragrance of a flower.

DAY 5 - SERVICE

I become quiet and attuned to my innerself. I feel my inner soul yearning for freedom and the experience of the Lord. My body, senses, mind, and intellect are tools to let my soul express itself.

I was put in the world for a specific mission. I accept and become aware of all my situations and predicaments in life. I use my total being to perform my duties spontaneously without ego or attachment. This is my dharma (duty).

Performance of dharma will purify me. I will be creative and perform my actions skillfully so I feel rejuvenated instead of tired. While my body and mind perform these actions, my heart is tuned to God.

I shall keep my eyes on the goal and use all necessary means without being attached to them.

I shall keep my attention in the present and will live and enjoy each moment at a time without ego, pride, or attachment to the results or rewards.

I shall make my work my worship. I shall serve all human beings with humility as God expresses Himself through all living beings.

I shall consider service as a privilege for self-purification.

DAY 6 - FREEDOM

As I become quiet, I experience the Self within my heart. I meditate on the omnipotent nature of the Self within. It is all powerful and always free from limitations of body and mind, time and space, cause and effect.

Liberation (Moksha) is the highest attainment of freedom. I become aware of the freedom of my soul which protects me against the illusions of the world (Maya).

As I direct my total being toward the divine Lord within me, my confusions, petty desires, hopes, and ambitions drop away.

As my attraction for the higher Self increases, bad habits fall away and positive disciplines come naturally without effort. These disciplines bring freedom.

Self is all pervading like ether. As I tune into the nature of this Self, I attract success in life from universal sources which provide me with abundance. I remain content and satisfied.

I gain greater freedom by giving, as giving is receiving. I feel greater freedom by surrendering my fears, guilts, worries, and ego. Thus, I feel weightlessness and freedom from burdens.

During the day I will recharge myself by tuning into my innerself to rise above limitations of the world. I shall realize that nothing is impossible for the omnipotent Self.

DAY 7 - PURITY

As I become quiet, I experience the presence of the higher Self. Self is ever pure and blissful. The world cannot contaminate it. The sun can be covered by clouds and a diamond can be covered by dirt. In the same way, the Self can be hidden behind impurities of body and mind, but It becomes visible as soon as the covers are removed.

I meditate on the luminous light of Self that destroys ignorance, doubts, and suffering.

I choose to fast one day a week to purify my body and to be aware that I don't live by bread alone, but with the divine love of God and Prana. If I choose to eat on this one day, I shall eat sparingly with full awareness of energy intake by eating and breathing.

I choose to purify my senses by resting them and abstaining from sights, sounds, reading, thinking, traveling, and other restless activities.

I choose to observe silence to preserve my mental energy and direct it toward God. If I choose to talk, I shall do so with full awareness and use only sweet and necessary words to preserve my energy of speech and mind. I shall express my love with pleasant gestures so that I shall not offend others by my silence.

If I choose to read, I shall read only scriptures and will do introspection to renew enthusiasm for my spiritual journey.

I shall purify my heart by letting go of hate, resentment, and fear, extending my love to everyone around me.

A map is only a guideline for a traveler. The rivers, bridges, roads, etc. on the map are only symbolically presented. Real experience is different. Scriptures and guidance of spiritual souls are only maps. One should travel the path himself for personal experience.

**

The world is a cosmic dream. Everyone and everything is a part of this dream. We realize this only when we wake up into transcendental reality through meditation. A dreamer's dream is real until he wakes up.

**

The world's reality has names, forms, causes and effects. Transcendental reality has only pure existence and essence of everything. Gold is the essence behind all golden ornaments.

**

Satsang mellows a person and loosens a stiff ego. Soaked beans cook more quickly than dried beans. A person with constant satsang matures in spiritual wisdom quickly.

**

An ignorant person enjoys the bliss of ignorance. As one awakens, the process produces suffering. When one becomes enlightened he enjoys the bliss of knowledge, which is permanent.

**

Meditation is introspection. If you are lost on a dark night in the countryside, you should look at the map to find out where you are and where you want to go, and set the right direction. Faster driving without direction will get you lost further and will disorient you. Restless running in life without introspection only produces confusion.

****

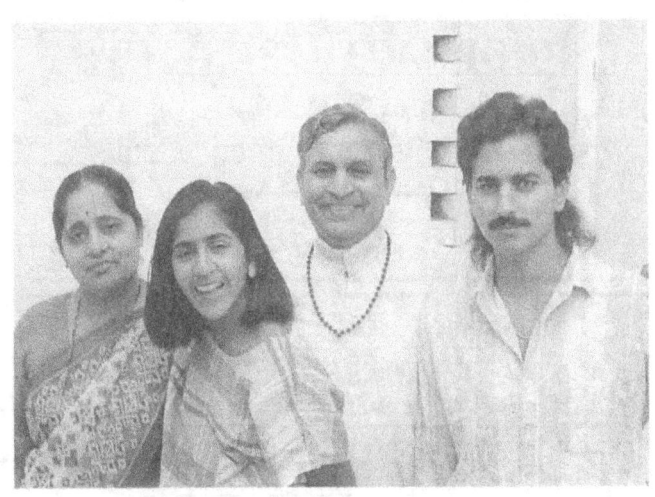

YOGI DESAI AND FAMILY 1987
Nayana (wife), Suchita (daughter) and Nipur (son)

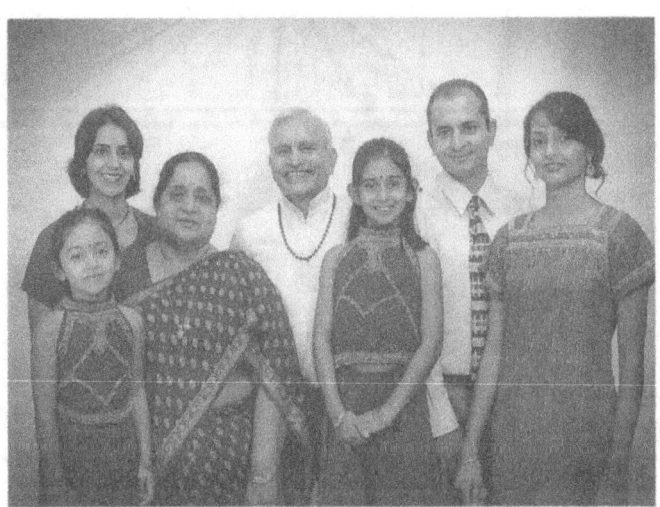

YOGI SHANTI DESAI AND FAMILY 2004
Kajal (daughter-in-law), Nisha 7, Maya 5 (grand daughters)

SHANTI YOGA INSTITUTE

CHIROPRACTIC SERVICES
by Nipur S. Desai, DC
Ocean Heights Chiropractic Center
2102 Ocean Heights Avenue,
Egg Harbor Township, NJ 08234
(609) 653-6624

MASSAGE THERAPIST
Suchita S. Desai
609-399-1974

YOGA RETREAT

- Yogic Vacation
- Instruction
- Consultation with Yogi Shanti Desai
- Seminars

943 Central Avenue
Ocean City, New Jersey 08226
(609) 399-1974

		52 To Somers Point		
		BUS		HAVEN
				WEST
	10th St.	9th St.	8th St.	ASBURY
To Cape May	Retreat		To Atlantic City (10 Miles)	CENTRAL
(30 Miles)				WESLEY
N				OCEAN
				ATLANTIC
	BOARDWALK			
	OCEAN			

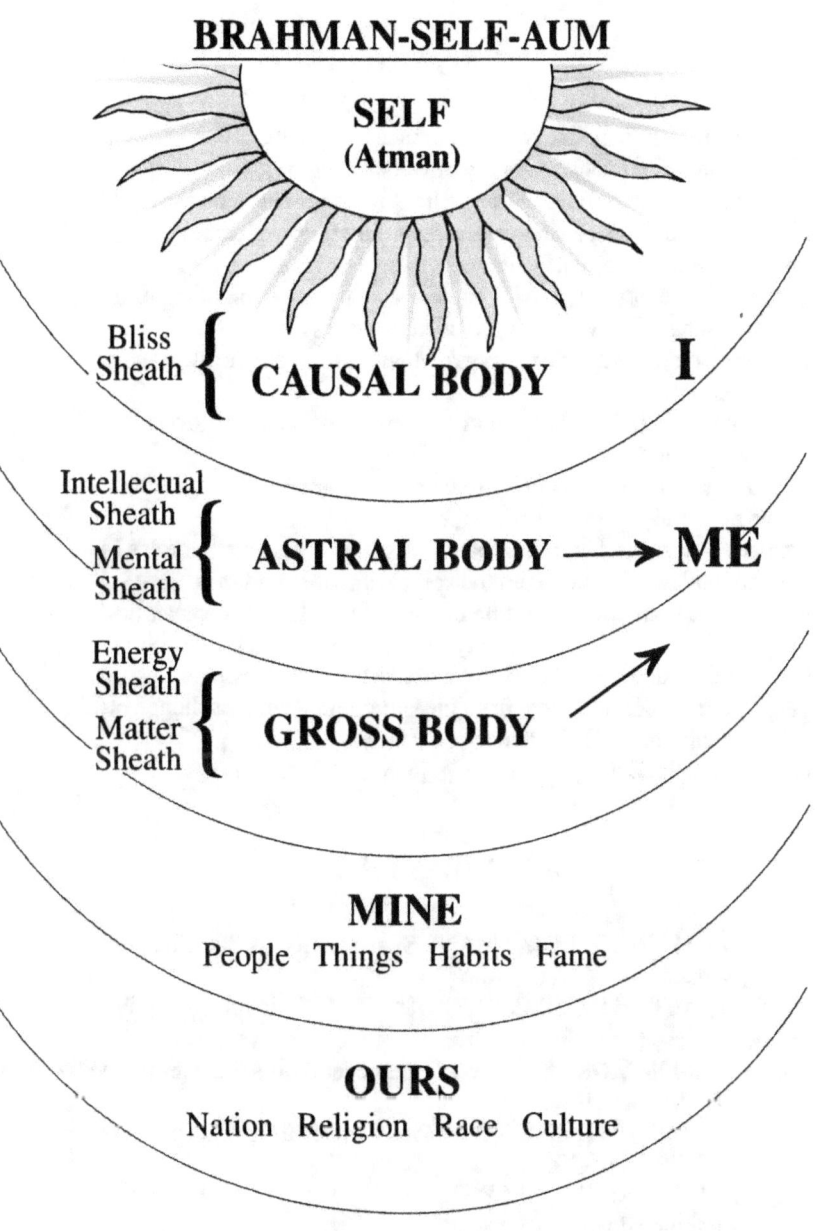

NEGATIONS

I have no race or nationality. Human race is my nationality.
I have no religion. Dharma is my universal religion.
I have no dogma or beliefs. Divine light removes my ignorance.
I have no family. All living creatures are my family members.
I have no home. The entire universe is my home.
I have no fame or power. All I have is a small reflection of the divine.
I own nothing. Everything is provided, as necessary, by the divine.
I possess no one. I am here to serve others for my purification and
    evolution.
I control nothing. I am only an instrument. Cosmic laws govern
    everything.
I rely on nothing and no one. I rely on divine grace and satsang.
I have no name. Name is just a label.
I am not father, brother, son, mother, or sister. These are the roles I play.
I am not male or female. I am the spirit without boundaries.
I am not the body. It is vibrating energy which changes constantly.
I am not the senses. They are only means of perceptions and actions.
I am not the mind. Mind does not exist. Mind is the changing waves
I am free from duality. Free from pleasure-pain, gain-loss, honor-insult.
I am not emotions. They change constantly.
I am not intellect. I rely on divine guidance and intuition.

AFFIRMATIONS

- ❖ I AM THE SELF (ATMAN): Spark of God as Sat, Chit and
  Anand.
- ❖ I AM THE BLISS CONSCIOUSNESS: Uninvolved passive
  witness to the drama of life
- ❖ I AM IMMORTAL: Never born, never dying. I am sustained by
  the divine energy.
- ❖ I HAVE NOTHING TO ATTAIN, NOTHING TO BE, NO-
  WHERE TO GO.
- ❖ I AM PERFECT, SELF SUFFICIENT, CONTENT: Need
  nothing added to life.
- ❖ I AM PERFECT AND FREE, HERE AND NOW: Nothing or
  nobody binds me.

ATMAN-BRAHMAN-JAGAT

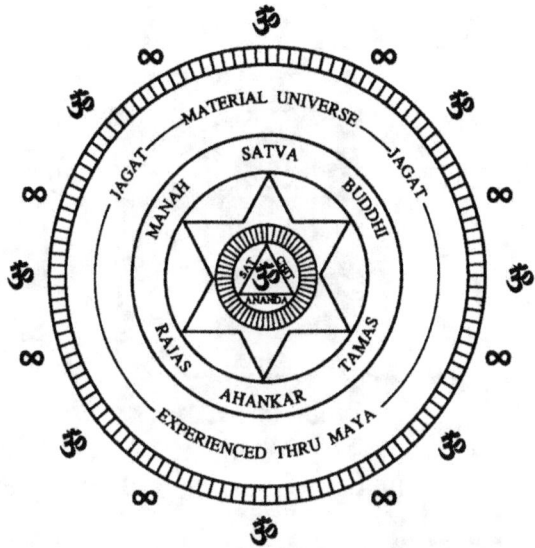

Brahman is omnipresent, absolute, ever expanding, without beginning or end. It is represented as infinity or Aum.

Atman is the reflection of Brahman, within everyone, and is represented as zero or void.

Jagat is Brahman experienced through the limitations of nature (Maya). It becomes the ephemeral universe (Jagat).

Jagat is the product of the two triangles of Maya.

1. Triangle of the subject - It is made of perceiving mind (Manah), discriminating mind (Buddhi) and I consciousness (Ahankar).

2. Triangle of the object - It is made of the three forces of nature (Gunas): balance (Satva), activity (Rajas), and inertia (Tamas).

Since the object and the subject are constantly changing, Jagat is impermanent (Mithya) or unreal (Asat). Brahman is an unchanging, constant reality (Sat).

Brahman is considered a macrocosm, while Atman is a microcosm. Both of them are beyond the grasp of the mind (subject) and the control of the three forces of nature (object). Both Infinity and Zero are transcendental and identical in nature.

Brahman = Infinity = Atman = Zero = Self = Aum

The purpose of meditation is to transcend the mind and to experience the self. In meditation, one either dissolves into zero or expands into infinity.

ENCYCLOPEDIA FOR LIVING
BY YOGI SHANTI DESAI

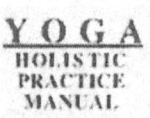
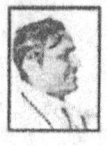
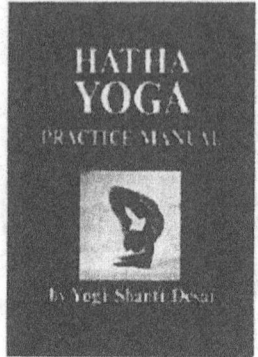
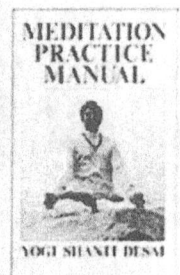

$14.00 $12.00 $10.00

Practice Manual 3 book set $30.00 (save $6)

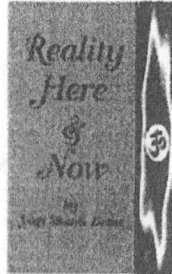
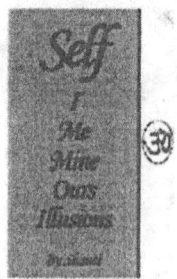
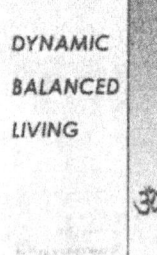

$8.00 $12.00 $3.00

Philosophy & Guidance 3 book set $18.00 (Save $5)
Or get all 6 books for $45.00

ADDITIONAL PRACTICE MATERIALS

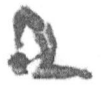
Video Tape
$18.00

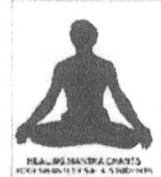
Mantra Chant
cassette tapes
volume 1 & 2
$13.00

www.ingramcontent.com/pod-product-compliance
Lightning Source LLC
Chambersburg PA
CBHW060240290526
45789CB00001B/124